Neuroleptic Syndrome and Related Conditions

Second Edition

MW00629184

Neuroleptic Malignant Syndrome and Related Conditions

Second Edition

Stephan C. Mann, M.D.

Associate Professor, Department of Psychiatry,
University of Pennsylvania School of Medicine, and
Department of Veterans Affairs Medical Center,
Philadelphia, Pennsylvania

Stanley N. Caroff, M.D.

Professor, Department of Psychiatry,
University of Pennsylvania School of Medicine, and
Department of Veterans Affairs Medical Center,
Philadelphia, Pennsylvania

Paul E. Keck Jr., M.D.

Vice Chairman for Research and Professor,
Departments of Psychiatry and Pharmacology,
University of Cincinnati School of Medicine, Cincinnati, Ohio

Arthur Lazarus, M.D., M.B.A.

Professor, Department of Psychiatry,
Drexel University College of Medicine, Philadelphia, Pennsylvania
Director and Regional Medical Research Specialist,
Pfizer Pharmaceutical Group, Prospect, Kentucky

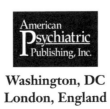

American Psychiatric Publishing, Inc.

Washington, DC
London, England

Note: The authors have worked to ensure that all information in this book is accurate at the time of publication and consistent with general psychiatric and medical standards, and that information concerning drug dosages, schedules, and routes of administration is accurate at the time of publication and consistent with standards set by the U.S. Food and Drug Administration and the general medical community. As medical research and practice continue to advance, however, therapeutic standards may change. Moreover, specific situations may require a specific therapeutic response not included in this book. For these reasons and because human and mechanical errors sometimes occur, we recommend that readers follow the advice of physicians directly involved in their care or the care of a member of their family.

Books published by American Psychiatric Publishing, Inc., represent the views and opinions of the individual authors and do not necessarily represent the policies and opinions of APPI or the American Psychiatric Association.

Copyright © 2003 American Psychiatric Publishing, Inc.
ALL RIGHTS RESERVED

Manufactured in the United States of America on acid-free paper
07 06 05 04 03   5 4 3 2 1
Second Edition

Typeset in Adobe's Janson Text and Berliner Grotesk

American Psychiatric Publishing, Inc.
1000 Wilson Boulevard, Suite 1825
Arlington, VA 22209-3901
www.appi.org

Library of Congress Cataloging-in-Publication Data
Neuroleptic malignant syndrome and related conditions / Stephan C. Mann . . . [et al.].—
2nd ed.
    p. ; cm.
  Rev. ed. of: Neuroleptic malignant syndrome and related conditions / Arthur Lazarus,
Stephan C. Mann, Stanley N. Caroff. c1989.
  Includes bibliographical references and index.
  ISBN 1-58562-011-4 (alk. paper)
    1. Neuroleptic malignant syndrome. 2. Antipsychotic drugs—Side effects. I. Mann,
Stephan C., 1948– II. Lazarus, Arthur, 1954– Neuroleptic malignant syndrome and
related conditions.
    [DNLM: 1. Neuroleptic Malignant Syndrome. 2. Antipsychotic Agents—adverse
effects. 3. Catatonia. 4. Heat Stroke. 5. Malignant Hyperthermia. 6. Serotonin Syndrome.
WL 307 N49423 2003]
RC394.N47 L38 2003
616.8—dc21

                                                                            2002027692

British Library Cataloguing in Publication Data
A CIP record is available from the British Library.

This book is lovingly dedicated to our wives,
Maureen, Rosalind, Susan, and Cheryl, and to our children.

Contents

Preface

The introduction of antipsychotic drugs in the mid-1950s revolutionized the treatment of schizophrenia and other psychotic disorders, allowing many patients in chronic hospital settings to return to the community. Although antipsychotics do not cure schizophrenia, they have decreased the disability and suffering associated with this disorder and have enabled many patients to enjoy more independent and productive lives. Shortly after antipsychotics came into clinical use, it became apparent that they had numerous undesirable side effects. Fortunately, most side effects are mild. Some rare side effects, however, are associated with significant discomfort, disability, or even death.

Neuroleptic malignant syndrome (NMS) was first described in France during early clinical trials of antipsychotics. However, it remained obscure and largely unrecognized in the English language literature until the 1980s. By 1986, more than 300 cases of NMS had been reported. Also in 1986, the term *neuroleptic malignant syndrome* was included as a specific medical heading in *Index Medicus*. However, in our work with NMS during this period, we found that most clinicians were unaware of or had only a limited appreciation of this disorder. Furthermore, the topic had been largely neglected in psychiatry texts of that era. "Reading up on NMS" meant culling the American and foreign literature and, at best, obtaining information in a piecemeal fashion. Yet, it seemed to us that investigators familiar with NMS were beginning to develop meaningful strategies for recognizing, diagnosing, and treating this disorder; these strategies could prove critical in avoiding a fatal outcome. It was in this context that we decided to write the first edition of *The Neuroleptic Malignant Syndrome and Related Conditions*, which was published in 1989.

In preparing the first edition of this book, we believed that it was essential to approach NMS as one of a group of related and, at times, clinically indistinguishable stress- and drug-induced hyperthermic syndromes encountered in medical and psychiatric practice. These syndromes included malignant (lethal) catatonia, antipsychotic drug–induced heat-stroke, and malignant hyperthermia (MH) of anesthesia. Furthermore, similar hyperthermic presentations could be induced by drugs other than neuroleptics such as stimulants, psychedelics, anticholinergics, lithium, tricyclic antidepressants, and monoamine oxidase inhibitors or occur during withdrawal from dopamine agonists, alcohol, or sedatives. We viewed an understanding of these related disorders as paramount not only in terms of differential diagnosis and development of management strategies but also as a critical source of comparative data relevant to common pathogenetic mechanisms.

Fourteen years have passed since the first edition of this book. Increasing recognition of NMS has resulted in the publication of hundreds of case reports and numerous reviews. The abundance of replicated clinical observations, including recent prospective studies of consecutive cases, has supported a more precise definition of NMS, clarified risk factors, stimulated interest in the related hyperthermic disorders, and provided insights into pathogenesis. We believe that enhanced recognition and improved management have reduced the incidence and mortality of NMS. However, because NMS occurs infrequently, individual practitioners still may have a limited appreciation of this disorder. Furthermore, the literature continues to reflect a lack of consensus on several key aspects of NMS, including its management, and clinicians often are baffled by the array of hyperthermic conditions that overlap with NMS and complicate the differential diagnosis. This lack of consensus among investigators coupled with the recent burgeoning data available served to underscore the need for a current and comprehensive review and prompted us to write the second edition of *Neuroleptic Malignant Syndrome and Related Conditions*.

Different opinions currently exist regarding the relation of NMS to the catatonic syndrome. Spurred in part by this debate, questions have been raised about the comparative efficacy of specific treatments for NMS. The relative advantage of dopamine agonists, benzodiazepines, dantrolene, or electroconvulsive therapy over each other or over supportive treatment alone remains unclear. Some investigators have begun to propose management guidelines individualized for each patient and based empirically on the character, duration, and severity of clinical signs and symptoms. In addition, with a better understanding of full-blown NMS, focus has begun to shift to milder, atypical, early, or suspected cases. Furthermore, the potential effect of the atypical antipsychotics on the incidence of NMS and the risk of causing recurrent episodes has yet to be adequately clarified.

The first edition contained an entire chapter devoted to MH. However, it has since become clear that despite remarkable clinical similarities, MH and NMS involve distinctly different pharmacological mechanisms.

Furthermore, other than being included in the differential diagnosis of NMS, MH is rarely encountered by psychiatrists. Accordingly, we now confine our discussion of MH to Chapter 1. Furthermore, the increase in clinical reports, academic interest, and controversy surrounding the NMS-like serotonin syndrome has led us to dedicate a separate chapter to this condition apart from other drug-induced hyperthermic disorders.

Each author of this second edition of *Neuroleptic Malignant Syndrome and Related Conditions* serves on the professional advisory council and as a hot-line consultant for the Neuroleptic Malignant Syndrome Information Service (NMSIS), a national project established in 1997 for disseminating information and accumulating data relating to NMS. On the hot line and at our booth at annual meetings of the American Psychiatric Association, each of us has been asked about the availability of a thorough, up-to-date reference on NMS. In addition, the overwhelming majority of psychiatrists who were surveyed by NMSIS indicated the need for more information on NMS. We hope that this second edition of *Neuroleptic Malignant Syndrome and Related Conditions* answers that need and provides psychiatrists and mental health professionals, primary care providers, neurologists, and other clinicians who deal with psychopharmacological agents with a current, balanced, and comprehensive synthesis of all the available data in this field. Furthermore, we hope to stimulate researchers to advance our knowledge of NMS through creative design of valid clinical trials and the development of reliable animal models.

Our sincere thanks go to Joanne Loguidice for her skillful secretarial assistance and manuscript preparation.

CHAPTER 1

Neuroleptic Malignant Syndrome

The introduction of antipsychotic drugs a half-century ago had a profound and enduring effect on the treatment of psychotic disorders. The safety and efficacy of these agents in treating psychosis have been well established. With the development of newer atypical antipsychotics in the last decade, the feasibility of achieving effective antipsychotic therapy that is relatively free of neurological complications appears ever closer to reality.

Neurological side effects produced by antipsychotic drugs are well known and, although often unpleasant and significant for the patient, are rarely life threatening. One notable exception is the neuroleptic malignant syndrome (NMS). Although its initial recognition and acceptance as a drug-induced syndrome were delayed, increasing awareness of NMS by clinicians resulted in numerous published case reports, clinical investigations, reviews, and meta-analyses. These studies have supported the development of standardized diagnostic criteria, clarified risk factors and treatment strategies, and shed light on the underlying pathogenesis of the syndrome. These findings have translated directly into better outcomes and reduced morbidity, mortality, and clinicians' liability. Furthermore, NMS has rekindled interest in classical hyperthermic disorders encountered in psychiatric practice. Thus, forthright acceptance and study of this iatrogenic syndrome have yielded new knowledge and enhanced the safety of managing severe psychotic conditions.

Despite these significant advances, there is a continuing need for study and education concerning NMS and related hyperthermic conditions. NMS is uncommon, and few clinicians are experienced in its management. The clinical manifestations of NMS are obscure to many practicing physicians, and the differential diagnosis may be difficult to delineate. In the absence of controlled trials, the treatment of NMS remains empirical and confusing to most practitioners. Fascinating questions remain concerning the pathogenesis of NMS and its relation to other hyperthermic disorders. NMS is still potentially life threatening if misdiagnosed, and this underscores the need for increased awareness of the diagnosis and management of this serious drug reaction.

🗐 Historical Background

The term *syndrome malin* had long been used in France as a nonspecific medical term referring to a fulminant, neurovegetative state that preceded collapse and death. As a purely descriptive term, *syndrome malin* had many etiologies. It was often associated with fever and fatal infectious processes. Delay and associates (1960) employed the term *syndrome malin des neuroleptiques* when similar alarming findings were observed in neuroleptic-treated patients: pallor, hyperthermia, and respiratory and psychomotor abnormalities.

The English translation of *syndrome malin des neuroleptiques*—"neuroleptic malignant syndrome"—first appeared in 1968. Delay and Deniker (1968) considered NMS "the most serious but also the rarest and least known of the complications of neuroleptic chemotherapy" (p. 258). It should be noted that what has been lost in translation and often misunderstood is that the syndrome, not the neuroleptic, is "malignant."

Prior to the 1960s, clinical descriptions of cases resembling NMS associated with phenothiazines were not formally diagnosed as NMS (Caroff 1980). In all of these cases, the adverse effects of neuroleptics were considered to be secondary to their actions on regulatory centers in the central nervous system (CNS). Interest in and increased awareness of febrile catatonic and parkinsonian states associated with antipsychotic administration were quite evident by the mid-1970s. By this time, NMS had been reported in France, Japan, and England. Several American researchers, cognizant of the French reports, also began to use the term *neuroleptic malignant syndrome* to describe similar cases in the United States (Meltzer 1973; Powers et al. 1976; Weinberger and Kelly 1977).

Caroff (1980) published a frequently cited review of NMS in English in 1980. He examined more than 60 cases described in the world literature at that time and suggested that NMS was seriously underrecognized and underdiagnosed. He used diagnostic criteria similar to those proposed by Delay and Deniker (1968) (i.e., hyperthermia, rigidity, altered consciousness, and autonomic instability) and cited reports that suggested that NMS may occur in as many as 0.5%–1% of neuroleptic-treated patients and may culminate in death in 20% of cases. In his survey of clinical material available at the time, Caroff (1980) also outlined demographic characteristics of affected patients and the major clinical features and course of NMS.

Consistent with earlier reports, the review by Caroff (1980) suggested that NMS could be distinguished from neuroleptic-related heatstroke and appeared to be similar to malignant hyperthermia (MH) and lethal catatonia. The association between these conditions and hyperthermic syndromes related to other drugs suggested that NMS may be the neuroleptic-induced subtype of a more generalized spectrum of hyperthermic disorders that could be induced in susceptible patients by a variety of pharmacological agents.

It is not clear why NMS received belated recognition in the United States. In this regard, one sees a parallel between NMS and tardive dyskinesia. Yet tardive dyskinesia generally takes years to develop, whereas NMS has a dramatic presentation and usually occurs during the early phase of treatment. It is disconcerting that despite the widespread use of antipsychotics, these two relatively severe reactions were not recognized earlier. Possible reasons for the belated recognition of NMS may involve the preponderance of early reports and reviews in diverse languages and the failure to distinguish signs and symptoms of NMS from idiopathic catatonic conditions, benign extrapyramidal reactions, and medical complications or medical illnesses that resemble NMS. The history of NMS is an object lesson in the need for clinical vigilance and postmarketing surveillance.

🗿 Epidemiology

Incidence

Although NMS is uncommon, the widespread use of neuroleptic drugs suggests that the absolute number of cases is significant (Caroff and Mann 1993; Caroff et al. 2001a). In a survey from Japan (S. Yamawaki et al. 1988, 1990b), two-thirds of facilities reported having experienced cases of NMS. A total of 1,666 suspected cases were reported.

A reasonable estimate of the incidence of NMS can be obtained by pooling the results of studies reporting the occurrence of NMS among large numbers of patients treated with antipsychotics at a particular center. This results in a figure of about 0.1%–0.2%, or 1 case of NMS in every

500–1,000 patients treated (Caroff and Mann 1993; Lazarus et al. 1989).
However, estimates of the risk have varied widely, ranging from 0.02%
to more than 3.0%. Incidence rates have varied depending on diagnostic
criteria, survey techniques, susceptibility of patients, clinical settings, and
prescribing practices. Most critically, the base denominator of patients
treated with antipsychotics is often estimated or derived from retrospective
data.

Some investigators have shown that the incidence rate of NMS may be
decreased by awareness and education of staff and conservative use of antipsychotics. For example, Gelenberg et al. (1988, 1989) reported only
1 NMS case (0.07%) in 1,470 patients during a 1-year period and no further cases among 1,450 patients treated during a second year of observation. They emphasized education of staff in recognizing and treating
incipient cases of NMS and conservative drug-dosing strategies. Keck and
colleagues (1987, 1991) reported 4 cases of NMS (0.15%) in 2,695 treated
patients in a prospective survey, which represented a decline from a prior
survey at the same center. They attributed the decline to early diagnosis
and risk reduction strategies.

Although the newer atypical antipsychotic drugs appear to spare the
extrapyramidal motor system, resulting in reduced liability for movement
disorders (Caroff et al. 2002), the incidence of NMS with these agents is
unclear (Caroff et al. 2000a). In centralized surveys, Sachdev et al. (1995)
reported a frequency of 3 cases of NMS (0.24%) in 1,250 patients receiving
clozapine, and Williams and MacPherson (1997) estimated the incidence
of NMS to be 9 (0.10%) in 9,000 clozapine-treated patients. In premarket-
ing trials, the manufacturer of quetiapine reported 2 cases of possible NMS
(0.08%) in 2,387 patients (Physicians' Desk Reference 2002). These figures
are similar to the incidence of NMS estimated to occur among patients
treated with typical antipsychotics.

In contrast, Kozaric-Kovacic et al. (1994) reported no cases of NMS in
866 episodes of treatment with clozapine, compared with 17 cases of NMS
(0.59%) in 2,897 treatment episodes involving haloperidol or fluphenazine,
a statistically significant difference. This is the only direct comparison
study showing a reduced incidence of NMS with an atypical drug compared with typical agents in a large patient sample.

Apart from data on overall incidence rates, several reports have indicated increased frequency or clustering of NMS cases at some sites, probably reflecting heightened awareness and case detection (Chopra et al.
1999; Destee et al. 1980; Fabre et al. 1977; Greenberg and Gujavarty 1985;
Harsch 1987; Huckle et al. 1993; H. Itoh et al. 1977; Janati and Webb
1986; Kimsey et al. 1983; Maling et al. 1988; Nicklason et al. 1991;
K. Thomas et al. 1993). Analyzing these data collectively from centers

around the world yields a mean ratio of 0.42 cases of NMS per month, or about five cases of suspected NMS encountered each year at an average representative medical center.

In summary, NMS appears to be uncommon, but a few cases are likely to be encountered annually in most medical centers. The incidence has been diminished at some centers by increasing awareness of and attention to proposed risk factors. The incidence and risks of NMS with newer, atypical antipsychotics are unclear but are probably reduced.

Risk Factors

As suggested by some investigators, it would be important to identify both susceptible patients who may be at risk for developing NMS and prescribing practices that may increase that risk. In fact, several small controlled studies have been conducted in an attempt to identify potential risk factors.

Age is not a helpful risk factor. Although NMS is reported often in young and middle-aged adults, for whom higher doses of antipsychotic drugs may be used, it has been reported in all age groups following administration of antipsychotics (Caroff and Mann 1988, 1993). The mean age of patients with NMS has been estimated to be about 40 years. In a national survey from Japan, 186 (89%) of 210 cases occurred in patients between ages 20 and 59 (S. Yamawaki et al. 1988). In one case-controlled study, age did not distinguish NMS patients from control subjects (Keck et al. 1989).

Although NMS can occur at any age, experience with the disorder in young children is limited. It has been suggested that young adult males (Caroff 1980), children (Shields and Bray 1976), and adolescents (Geller and Greydanus 1979) are at risk for NMS. Silva et al. (1999) reviewed the literature on NMS in children and adolescents and found 77 cases in patients ranging from 0.9 to 18 years of age. However, only 10 patients were younger than 11 years, and the incidence of reports increased with age, probably reflecting the lower rate of drug exposure in young children. In a fascinating review of Reye's syndrome in children, Casteels-Van Daele et al. (2000) raised the possibility that early studies of this disorder may have underestimated the side effects of phenothiazines used as antiemetics and that some of these cases actually may have been examples of NMS before it was widely recognized.

Like age, sex is not a meaningful risk factor for NMS, with studies reporting NMS more common in men, more common in women, or about equal between sexes (Caroff and Mann 1993; Deng et al. 1990; Keck et al. 1989; Tsutsumi et al. 1994).

The worldwide occurrence of NMS suggests that environmental factors do not play a primary role in causing the syndrome. Although Singh

(1984) claimed that reports of NMS were more frequent from countries with hot climates, based on the author's experience with a case that may have been heatstroke rather than NMS, NMS has occurred with ambient temperatures as low as 8.5°C (Schrader 1982). Moreover, analyses (Caroff and Mann 1988; Shalev et al. 1986) of the occurrence of NMS cases by month showed that NMS was not associated with hot summer months and that it occurred throughout the seasons. However, this does not preclude the possibility that high ambient heat and humidity may contribute to thermoregulatory dysfunction in a patient at risk for NMS (Shalev et al. 1988). Antipsychotic drugs interfere with central thermoregulation and, particularly in combination with anticholinergic drugs that inhibit sweating, can contribute to the development of heatstroke in a hot environment. However, heatstroke can be distinguished from NMS, as discussed later in this chapter in the "Differential Diagnosis" section.

NMS is not specific to any neuropsychiatric diagnosis. It has been reported to occur in patients receiving antipsychotic drugs for diverse neuropsychiatric disorders, as well as in medical patients with normal brain function who received neuroleptic drugs as antiemetics or sedatives (Caroff et al. 2001c; Moyes 1973; Patel and Bristow 1987). Caroff et al. (2001c) reviewed the literature and found 28 cases of NMS in surgical patients who received antipsychotics for behavioral control or neuroleptics for sedation and antiemesis. Surgical patients with histories of substance abuse, traumatic head injury, or neuropsychiatric disorders appeared to be particularly susceptible, but patients with no evidence of brain dysfunction also developed NMS.

Nevertheless, certain disorders may heighten the risk of NMS. Several authors have proposed that patients with schizophrenia (Shalev and Munitz 1986; S. Yamawaki et al. 1990b), mood disorders (Addonizio et al. 1986; Hermesh et al. 1992; Lazarus et al. 1989; Pearlman 1986; Rosebush and Stewart 1989), or organic brain disorders (Caroff 1980; Delay and Deniker 1968; Vincent et al. 1986) may be at risk for NMS. Patients with organic brain disease at risk for NMS have included those with underlying encephalitis (Caroff et al. 1998b, 2001b) and congenital and developmental disorders.

Patients with substance abuse or dependence may be at risk. In particular, alcoholic patients may have a lower threshold of resistance to neurotoxic side effects of antipsychotic drugs (Lutz 1976) and hence may be more susceptible to NMS. Alcoholism was diagnosed in 8% of NMS patients in one review (Levenson 1985). A particularly vulnerable time to develop NMS may be during acute withdrawal from alcohol or CNS depressant drugs (Burch and Downs 1987) when neurological status and thermoregulatory and autonomic mechanisms are already compromised.

Of particular significance are the reports by D.A.C. White and Robins (1991, 2000) that patients with preexisting idiopathic or antipsychotic-induced catatonia may be at risk for developing NMS when treatment with antipsychotics is initiated or continued. These findings are consistent with the conceptualization of NMS as a more fulminant form of catatonia.

Unfortunately, differences in diagnostic criteria of the underlying disorders, the rarity of NMS cases, variability in the use of psychotropic drugs, and the scarcity of large controlled trials limit conclusions on the relative susceptibility of diagnostic categories. There is a small but finite risk of developing NMS in any patient whenever neuroleptics or antipsychotics are prescribed.

Across many clinical reports and controlled studies, consistent evidence now indicates that systemic and metabolic factors, including agitation, exhaustion, and dehydration, may increase the risk for NMS. For example, H. Itoh et al. (1977) reported that physical exhaustion and dehydration preceded the onset of NMS in all 14 patients in their series. Harsch (1987) found dehydration in eight of nine NMS patients before the onset of the syndrome. In a case-controlled study, Keck et al. (1989) reported that agitation and dehydration were significantly associated with NMS. These findings have been consistently replicated by other investigators (Berardi et al. 1998; Naganuma and Fujii 1994; Rosebush and Stewart 1989; Sachdev et al. 1997; Tsutsumi et al. 1994). However, it should be noted that it is difficult to distinguish between dehydration as a preceding risk factor and dehydration as a result of fluid losses that occur during NMS. It also may be true that patients with comorbid medical or neurological illnesses that impair cardiovascular function and thermoregulation may be at higher risk for developing NMS and for a poorer outcome following NMS (Chopra et al. 1999).

Intuitively, patients with preexisting known or subclinical abnormalities in central brain dopamine activity or receptor function may constitute a high-risk group. This is exemplified by the development of NMS-like syndromes in association with various extrapyramidal disorders, including Parkinson's disease (see Chapter 4), Huntington's disease (Burke et al. 1981), Wilson's disease (Kontaxakis et al. 1988), striatonigral degeneration (Gibb 1988), and tardive dyskinesia or dystonia (Haggerty et al. 1987; Harris et al. 1987).

Because iron may play an integral role in central dopamine receptor function, Rosebush and colleagues (Rosebush and Mazurek 1991; Rosebush and Stewart 1989) measured serum iron levels in NMS patients and found a reduced level that appeared to be state specific in many patients. J.W.Y. Lee (1998) and Carroll and Goforth (1995) reported that patients with catatonia and low serum iron levels may be more likely to develop

NMS after treatment with antipsychotics. However, the reliability of serum iron concentrations as a diagnostic marker or risk factor for NMS has not been sufficiently investigated or replicated in all studies (E. Turner and Reddy 1991; Weller and Kornhuber 1993).

Studies of the familial occurrence or genetic markers of NMS have received limited attention. Deuschl et al. (1987) reported the occurrence of NMS in twin brothers with schizophrenia. Otani et al. (1991) reported episodes of NMS in a mother and two daughters, all of whom had catatonic schizophrenia, and speculated that this family shared a vulnerability in central dopaminergic systems. These findings are consistent with reports of the familial occurrence of idiopathic lethal catatonia by Stauder (1934) and others and more recent investigations of genetic mechanisms in catatonic disorders.

Lazarus et al. (1991) diagnosed NMS in a retarded patient with an inverted duplication of chromosome 5. Rubio-Gozalbo et al. (2001) reported the occurrence of NMS in a patient with X-linked cerebral adrenoleuko-dystrophy, a progressive metabolic disease affecting the nervous system. Manor et al. (1997) reported the occurrence of NMS in two siblings with gangliosidosis, type 2. The occurrence of NMS in these patients may reflect the nonspecific higher risk in patients with underlying organic brain disease rather than linkage with a specific genetic defect.

MH of anesthesia is another NMS-like drug-induced hyperthermic syndrome (Lazarus et al. 1989). MH is considered to be an autosomal dominant pharmacogenetic disorder involving a membrane-related defect in calcium sequestration in skeletal muscle. More than 50% of families show linkage of the MH phenotype to the gene encoding the skeletal muscle ryanodine receptor (RYR1) on chromosome 19, and more than 20 mutations have been described (Jurkat-Rott et al. 2000). To test the linkage of NMS susceptibility with mutations in the RYR1 gene, Miyatake et al. (1996) screened for 6 mutations in 10 patients who had NMS. Although they found none of the 6 mutations in the NMS patients, a mutation was detected in a control patient who had creatine phosphokinase (CPK) elevations during antipsychotic drug treatment. The negative findings in the NMS patients are consistent with data from family studies (Hermesh et al. 1988) and in vitro testing (Adnet and Krivosic-Horber 1990; Caroff et al. 1994a, 1994b), which indicate that NMS patients do not share a genetic defect with MH patients.

Attempts to identify patients at risk also have included studies of genetic markers in enzyme systems and neurotransmitter receptor structure. Iwahashi (1994) first reported a mutation in the cytochrome P450 2D6 (CYP2D6) gene in an elderly woman with NMS, and Kawanishi et al. (1998b) also reported mutations in two patients with NMS. However, larger controlled studies by these and other groups failed to confirm an association between NMS and CYP2D6 polymorphism (Iwahashi et al. 1999; Kawanishi et al. 2000; Ueno et al. 1996).

In 1995, Ram et al. reported on an analysis of the D_2 dopamine receptor gene in 12 patients with NMS, including a mother-daughter pair, but found a missense variation in only 1 patient. Kawanishi et al. (1998a) screened for polymorphisms in the serotonin type 1A ($5\text{-}HT_{1A}$) and serotonin type 2A ($5\text{-}HT_{2A}$) receptor genes among 29 patients previously diagnosed with NMS as compared with schizophrenic patients and healthy control subjects. They found no polymorphisms in these receptor genes that could serve as factors determining susceptibility to NMS. In contrast, Suzuki et al. (2001) reported a significantly higher frequency of the *Taq*I A_1 allele in the D_2 dopamine receptor gene of 15 patients with NMS compared with 138 patients with schizophrenia alone. The A_1 allele has been associated with diminished dopaminergic activity. If these findings can be replicated, they would suggest that the *Taq*I A polymorphism of the D_2 dopamine receptor gene may be associated with the predisposition to develop NMS.

Pharmacological and treatment variables also have been examined as risk factors for NMS (Caroff and Mann 1993). Approximately 17% of NMS patients reported a similar episode during prior treatment with antipsychotics (Caroff and Mann 1988; S. Yamawaki et al. 1988). Caroff and Mann (1988) also found that about 30% of NMS patients were at risk for future episodes or rechallenge with antipsychotic drugs. Similarly, Rosebush et al. (1989) found that 5 (33%) of 15 patients who had recovered from NMS developed at least one subsequent episode when rechallenged. These findings strongly imply that a history of a prior episode is a significant risk factor for a recurrent episode.

Virtually all classes of drugs that block D_2 dopamine receptors have been associated with NMS. In approximately one-third of reported cases, patients received more than one antipsychotic, making it difficult to distinguish the effects of individual drugs (Addonizio et al. 1987; Kurlan et al. 1984). However, most cases of NMS have been reported in patients receiving high-potency antipsychotics. Haloperidol has been implicated in nearly half of the reported cases and is the sole triggering agent in 28% of cases (Caroff and Mann 1988; S. Yamawaki et al. 1988). This observation has led many investigators to conclude that patients receiving high-potency neuroleptics are at increased risk for developing NMS. Alternative explanations may be possible, however, because high-potency neuroleptics may be prescribed more frequently and at higher milligram-equivalent dosages than low-potency neuroleptics (Baldessarini 1985). Also, high-potency antipsychotics may be more likely to be given to medically ill or young acutely psychotic patients who may be at higher risk for developing NMS (Caroff 1980; Levenson 1985). However, NMS may be caused by low-potency drugs and even atypical agents such as reserpine (Haggerty et al. 1987) and the newer antipsychotic agents (Caroff et al. 2000a).

Expectations were raised that the newer antipsychotics, with reduced D_2 receptor affinity and effects on other neurotransmitter systems that may mitigate extrapyramidal dysfunction, would reduce the incidence of NMS. Although the risk with these agents may be diminished, cases of NMS have been reported. Available data suggest that the incidence of NMS with atypical drugs may be the same as or less than with typical antipsychotics (Kozaric-Kovacic et al. 1994; Sachdev et al. 1995; Williams and MacPherson 1997). However, reports of NMS with atypical agents may be inflated because of the rush to report cases with new drugs and because patients switched to atypical agents may be more susceptible to NMS and drug intolerant in general (Caroff et al. 2000a).

Sachdev et al. (1995) concluded that NMS does occur with clozapine but may present with fewer and milder symptoms. Hasan and Buckley (1998) concurred that NMS may develop with clozapine and risperidone but not necessarily in atypical forms. Caroff et al. (2000a) examined cases from the literature and from the Neuroleptic Malignant Syndrome Information Service database and found that NMS as defined by diagnostic criteria did occur with atypical drugs and that extreme temperatures were less frequently observed than in cases of NMS triggered by typical drugs. Only NMS associated with clozapine had significantly reduced signs of rigidity and tremor. However, the question of whether atypical drugs are more likely to produce milder or atypical forms of NMS is rendered moot by the fact that the presentation of NMS often has been heterogeneous even with typical agents. In addition, reports of milder or partial forms of NMS have become more common because awareness of the diagnosis has increased such that cases are recognized and treated earlier.

The adverse effects of drugs with neuroleptic properties used in nonpsychiatric settings are often neglected and may not be recognized by other clinicians. This is true for cases of NMS as well. There have been many reports of NMS, including several deaths in patients treated with neuroleptic drugs for emesis (prochlorperazine), peristalsis (metoclopramide), anesthesia (droperidol), and sedation (promethazine). Caroff et al. (2001c) reported 28 case reports of NMS in the perioperative setting. Haloperidol, used in the treatment of agitation and delirium, was implicated in half the cases, whereas other neuroleptics accounted for the rest.

Data on dosage indicate that NMS is not a result of overdosage and occurs within the therapeutic range (Caroff and Mann 1988, 1993). Studies of recurrence of NMS after rechallenge have been inconsistent as to whether potency or dosage correlates with NMS. Caroff and Mann (1988) and Shalev and Munitz (1986) found that high-potency agents increased the risk, whereas in a prospective series of cases, Rosebush et al. (1989) found no relation between potency or dosage and recurrence of NMS.

Shalev and Munitz (1986) further proposed that the loading rate of neuroleptics in treating psychosis, rather than total dosage, is a key factor. In addition, perhaps related to the rate of loading (Shalev and Munitz 1986), the intramuscular and intravenous routes of administration seem to potentiate the development of NMS (H. Itoh et al. 1977). Kirkpatrick and Edelsohn (1985) found that NMS was correlated with high doses of neuroleptics, rather than rate of increase, although the validity of their results was questioned by Pearlman (1986). Neuroleptic blood levels, when measured, have been reported within normal limits (Lazarus 1985c; Lazarus et al. 1989).

More recently, most studies of risk factors, including some prospective controlled series, have supported the possibility that higher doses of high-potency antipsychotics administered at rapid rates of increase, particularly in parenteral forms, may be associated with an increased risk of NMS (Berardi et al. 1998; Chopra et al. 1999; Hermesh et al. 1992; Keck et al. 1989; Naganuma and Fujii 1994; Sachdev et al. 1997; Tsutsumi et al. 1994). However, this has not been confirmed in all studies (Deng et al. 1990; Rosebush and Stewart 1989), and it must be recognized that NMS has occurred even after a single low dose of an antipsychotic in susceptible individuals (Aisen and Lawlor 1992). Nevertheless, these findings support the benefits of conservative dosing practices and the hazards of rapid neuroleptization in psychotic patients.

Some investigators (Allan and White 1972; Caroff 1980; Grunhaus et al. 1979) have pointed out potential dangers for patients who develop NMS while receiving depot neuroleptics. All six cases of NMS reported by Kimsey et al. (1983) involved the administration of fluphenazine decanoate. Caroff's 1980 review indicated that long-acting fluphenazine compounds were associated with increased mortality in NMS, perhaps because the long half-life of these agents results in greater duration of exposure to the risk of medical complications. Pearlman (1986) confirmed the longer duration and morbidity of NMS with depot neuroleptics but not an increased mortality. Deng et al. (1990) compared treatment data on 12 NMS patients and 102 control patients. Although no differences were found between groups in the mean dosages of neuroleptics used, they found that NMS patients treated with intramuscular fluphenazine decanoate, a long-acting neuroleptic, had 3 times the rate of NMS, which rose to 10 times the rate when fluphenazine decanoate was administered without antiparkinsonian agents. This effect was not observed by Keck et al. (1989) but was supported by

Chopra et al. (1999). Although at present, evidence is not conclusive for increased incidence or mortality from NMS in relation to treatment with depot drugs, it would seem prudent to monitor the use of long-acting neuroleptics carefully in view of the probable longer duration and morbidity of NMS secondary to these drugs.

Another potential risk factor for NMS may relate to the switching, discontinuation, or restarting of antipsychotic drugs (Caroff et al. 2000a). The period after discontinuation of antipsychotic drugs may represent a time of relative instability in dopaminergic systems such that reintroduction of D_2 receptor blockade may precipitate NMS. NMS has been reported shortly after discontinuation of antipsychotics and frequently after antipsychotics were switched or restarted.

More than half of the cases of NMS involve the concomitant administration of medication other than neuroleptics (e.g., lithium carbonate, tricyclic antidepressants, antiparkinsonian medications, and benzodiazepines) (Caroff and Mann 1988, 1993). Whether these drugs offer some prophylactic advantage or, on the contrary, predispose to NMS cannot be answered as yet based on the limited data now available. However, evidence derived from cases of neuroleptic-related heatstroke strongly suggests a contributory role of anticholinergics in impairing heat loss, such that administration of anticholinergics may be disadvantageous in patients with high temperature in NMS. In contrast, Keck et al. (1989) and Deng et al. (1990) found no significant differences in the use of any concomitant drugs between small groups of NMS patients and neuroleptic-treated control subjects.

Primeau et al. (1987) postulated that poorly controlled extrapyramidal symptoms in neuroleptic-treated patients may be a risk factor for NMS. They reported that a change to a less potent anticholinergic drug (diphenhydramine) apparently precipitated NMS in three patients receiving haloperidol. In a similar report (Merriam 1987), NMS was precipitated by the apparent loss of cholinergic blockade consequent to a reduction in imipramine dose. These reports suggest that more active attempts to control or prevent extrapyramidal symptoms by using antiparkinsonian drugs may be beneficial in preventing NMS, as suggested by Levinson and Simpson (1986). However, particularly in view of clinical data showing a failure of antiparkinsonian anticholinergics to prevent or treat symptoms of NMS, it is possible that resistant extrapyramidal symptoms may herald NMS and could indicate the need for recognition and management of NMS.

In summary, no proven reliable risk factors outweigh the benefits of antipsychotic therapy in a given patient. Evidence is accumulating, however, to support catatonia, basal ganglia dysfunction, psychomotor agitation, dehydration, previous episodes of NMS, the rate of increase of neuroleptic dosage, and the use of parenteral medication as potential risk factors. It is difficult to demonstrate the significance of specific variables because the numbers of patients are small in any one study, control data are often lacking, and the variables may be interrelated or act synergistically. Furthermore, it is very difficult to develop reliable risk factors to predict the occurrence of a rare phenomenon such as NMS in a given population. Although statistical significance for some factors (e.g., agitation, parenteral injections) can be shown in small case-control studies, these variables are so common in the population of psychotic patients receiving treatment that excessive reliance on them would lead to a gross overestimation of the risk of NMS, numerous false-positive results, and the unnecessary withholding of effective antipsychotic therapy with potentially dire consequences.

🗿 Clinical Characteristics

Early Signs

Apart from identifying patients at risk, the identification of prodromal or early signs of NMS would be useful in facilitating intervention and aborting incipient episodes. At times, NMS may develop explosively and progress within hours, thus precluding recognition of early signs. But more commonly, NMS develops insidiously over days and is preceded by neurological and autonomic signs that are refractory to conventional measures.

Signs that may precede NMS include unexpected changes in mental status, particularly obtundation or new-onset catatonia; episodic tachycardia, tachypnea, or hypertension; dysarthria, dysphagia, diaphoresis, sialorrhea, incontinence, low-grade temperature elevations, rigidity, myoclonus, tremor, or other extrapyramidal signs unresponsive to antiparkinsonian agents; and unexplained elevations in serum CPK. However, these signs are nonspecific, do not necessarily progress to NMS, and do not invariably precede the syndrome. As a general rule, the diagnosis of NMS should be entertained if a patient unexpectedly appears to deteriorate neurologically in association with antipsychotic drug treatment.

Several investigators have proposed that autonomic, mental status, and extrapyramidal symptoms preceded other signs of NMS and that hyperthermia and hypermetabolism were relatively late developments that reflected the culmination of pathophysiological processes (Addonizio et al. 1987; Modestin et al. 1992; Velamoor et al. 1990). Velamoor et al. (1994, 1995) analyzed the pattern of symptom development in 153 clinical reports in the literature in which the chronology of symptom development was described. They found that neurological signs or mental status changes preceded systemic signs of NMS in 83.6% of cases. Mental status changes or muscle rigidity constituted the initial signs of the disorder in 82.3% of cases in which a single presenting sign could be ascertained. These findings of a predictable pattern in the early evaluation of symptoms are important in that unexpected mental status and extrapyramidal dysfunction may herald the onset of NMS. In addition, they reinforce the notion that NMS is triggered by the effects of antipsychotics on the CNS, which secondarily result in a systemic, hypermetabolic syndrome.

Clinical Signs and Symptoms

Patients with classic features of NMS have been described as presenting in a "hypothalamic," "adrenergic," "hypodopaminergic," or "parkinsonian" crisis, with evidence of hypermetabolism and increased oxygen consumption (May et al. 1983).

Hyperthermia usually develops as a late manifestation of the full-blown syndrome. Temperatures in excess of the 42°C limit of conventional thermometers have been reported. Hyperthermia is considered by many to be the most distinguishing feature of NMS, setting it apart from other neuroleptic-related conditions with varying combinations of extrapyramidal, autonomic, and neuropsychiatric dysfunction. Possible sources of hyperthermia in NMS include neuroleptic-induced inhibition of central dopaminergic thermoregulatory mechanisms mediating heat loss and increased heat production derived from neuroleptic effects on skeletal muscle tone and metabolism. Gurrera and Chang (1996) studied 46 episodes of NMS and reported a unique loss of integrated thermoeffector activity and coordination in these patients. Febrile medical complications of NMS, such as infection, dehydration, electrolyte imbalance, pulmonary embolus, atelectasis, rhabdomyolysis, and seizures, may secondarily contribute to elevated temperatures (Levinson and Simpson 1986) but do not explain the development of hyperthermia in most cases (Addonizio et al. 1987; Caroff and Mann 1988).

Hyperthermia associated with profuse sweating occurs in 98% of reported NMS cases, exceeding 38°C in 87% and 40°C in 40% (Caroff and Mann 1988; Caroff et al. 1991). Extreme hyperthermia may predispose to complications, including irreversible cerebellar or other brain damage, if not reduced immediately.

Muscle rigidity, hypertonicity, or unresponsiveness to antiparkinsonian agents is an early and characteristic sign of NMS and in combination with hyperthermia helps to differentiate the syndrome from other conditions. Generalized rigidity, described as "lead-pipe" in its most severe form, is reported in 97% of NMS cases and is associated with myonecrosis (Caroff and Mann 1988). Cogwheeling may or may not be present. Additional parkinsonian features such as tremor, sialorrhea, hypomimia, bradykinesia, and festinating gait may be present. Tremors are frequent, generalized, symmetrical, and impressive. Other neurological signs may include dystonia, chorea, trismus, dyskinesia, myoclonus, opisthotonos, oculogyric crises, opsoclonus, blepharospasm, dysarthria, dysphagia, abnormal reflexes, posturing, nystagmus, and ocular flutter (Kurlan et al. 1984). NMS may occur without evidence of severe muscle rigidity or other extrapyramidal signs if patients are simultaneously receiving skeletal muscle relaxants (Caroff et al. 2001c; Rogers and Stoudemire 1988), which is an important feature that distinguishes NMS from MH.

Changes in mental status have been reported in 97% of cases (Caroff and Mann 1988; Caroff et al. 1991). Manifestations include clouding of consciousness that varies from stupor to coma, delirium, and the development of catatonic features. The classic NMS patient is alert but appears dazed and mute, representing catatonia or akinetic mutism. Some patients continue to have periods of agitation during NMS, requiring sedation with benzodiazepines or physical restraints. The autonomic nervous system disturbances in NMS—tachycardia, tachypnea, profuse diaphoresis, labile blood pressure, urinary incontinence, and pallor—may be seen at any time and may provide an early clue to recognizing NMS. Autonomic activation and instability, manifested by sinus tachycardia (88%) or oscillations of blood pressure (61%), have been reported in 95% of cases (Caroff and Mann 1988). Moderate to severe respiratory distress and tachypnea, which may result from metabolic acidosis, hyperthermia, chest-wall restriction, aspiration pneumonia, or pulmonary emboli, may be observed in 31% of cases (S. Yamawaki et al. 1988, 1990b) and may lead to respiratory arrest.

Laboratory Abnormalities

Several clinical laboratory abnormalities are commonly reported in NMS, but most are nonspecific or reflect complications of the syndrome. Nevertheless, a comprehensive laboratory investigation is essential to rule out other causes of hyperthermia. Rhabdomyolysis or myonecrosis may result in markedly increased levels of serum CPK and myoglobinuria. CPK elevations may occur in up to 95% of NMS cases (Caroff and Mann 1988), reaching as high as 2,000 times normal values in some cases. More commonly, modest or equivocal elevations occur, which cannot be distinguished from the effects of nonspecific factors (e.g., agitation and injections). Serum aldolase also may be elevated, along with other serum enzymes (transaminases, lactic dehydrogenase), which are also released from damaged skeletal muscle cells but are often mistakenly attributed to liver damage. In contrast, elevations in hepatic bilirubin or alkaline phosphatase have not been reported to occur in NMS. Myoglobinuria was reported in 67% of the cases of NMS in which urine was tested (Caroff et al. 1991).

These findings support the frequent occurrence of muscle necrosis in NMS, which stems from rigidity, hyperthermia, and ischemia and may result in acute renal failure. Direct myotoxicity of neuroleptics remains controversial. Because factors such as agitation or intramuscular injections may contribute to elevations in CPK, the diagnostic value of serum enzymes has been questioned. However, measurement of CPK remains important as a measure of severity and the risk of renal failure.

Other common findings include a nonspecific leukocytosis with or without a left shift in 98% of cases and metabolic acidosis or hypoxia on blood-gas analysis in 75% of cases examined (Caroff and Mann 1988; Caroff et al. 1991). Findings indicative of disseminated intravascular coagulation—such as increased prothrombin time and activated partial thromboplastin time, increased fibrin split products, and decreased platelets— have been reported in several cases (Lazarus et al. 1989). Peripheral thrombophlebitis and pulmonary embolization also have been reported.

Cases of NMS have been reported in association with hyperglycemia and both hyponatremia and hypernatremia (Lazarus et al. 1989). These alterations in sodium may not have significance apart from the profound fluid and electrolyte disturbances that may develop in NMS, although some investigators have proposed diabetes, hyponatremia, or inappropriate antidiuretic hormone secretion as precipitating factors in NMS.

Low serum iron has been observed during NMS and has been proposed as a state-related marker for NMS (J.W.Y. Lee 1998; Rosebush and Mazurek 1991; Rosebush and Stewart 1989). However, low iron has not been observed in all cases (Weller and Kornhuber 1993) and, as is true for other laboratory abnormalities during NMS, may represent the nonspecific effects of an acute-phase reaction (E. Turner and Reddy 1991).

Increased peripheral levels of monoamines and their metabolites have been reported in NMS and undoubtedly reflect the autonomic activation or "adrenergic crisis" that occurs as part of NMS (Feibel and Schiffer 1981; Schibuk and Schachter 1986). Recently, Spivak et al. (2000) reported finding reduced circulating dopamine and elevated epinephrine and serotonin concentrations in platelet-poor plasma obtained from eight NMS patients. These results were interpreted as reflecting a reduction in dopaminergic activity and an increase in adrenergic and serotoninergic activity in the acute NMS state.

Electroencephalographic examination findings may be abnormal in about 50% of NMS cases, indicating generalized, nonspecific slowing consistent with encephalopathy in most instances.

Viewed as a diagnosis of exclusion, NMS can be supported only when other disorders are ruled out. Normal computerized tomographic scans of the head have been obtained in 95% of cases reported in the literature (Caroff and Mann 1988). The few abnormal scans showed evidence of pre-existing pathology (e.g., atrophy or trauma). Similarly, examination of cerebrospinal fluid (CSF) was normal in 95% of cases (Caroff and Mann 1988). These results suggest that it is unlikely that a central organic etiology, unrelated to drug treatment, is responsible for the clinical manifestations of NMS in most cases.

In 75 cases reported between 1980 and 1987 in which the results of evaluation for sepsis were specified, multiple cultures of body fluids failed to identify an organism that could account for the syndrome (Caroff and Mann 1988). Thus, most reported cases of NMS are not infectious in origin. However, cultures may be positive in cases secondarily complicated by infection. In addition, it may be difficult to distinguish primary from secondary infections, and patients with preexisting infections such as encephalitis may be at risk for NMS (Caroff et al. 1998b, 2001b).

🔌 Diagnostic Criteria

The consistent clinical and laboratory features reported in hundreds of case reports and reviews of NMS have enabled several groups to develop standardized diagnostic criteria. Although there are differences, most sets of criteria include comparable major components. Levenson (1985) suggested that the presence of three major manifestations (fever, rigidity, and increased CPK) or two major and four of six minor manifestations (tachycardia, abnormal blood pressure, tachypnea, altered consciousness, diaphoresis, and leukocytosis) indicated a high probability of NMS if supported by the clinical history. Levenson's criteria may be highly sensitive and inclusive but less specific because of the possibility of diagnosing NMS in the absence of rigidity and the weight given to the nonspecific finding of CPK elevation (S.D. Roth et al. 1986).

Pope et al. (1986) suggested that NMS was diagnosable based on hyperthermia, severe extrapyramidal symptoms, and autonomic dysfunction and that altered mental status, leukocytosis, and elevated CPK could be used retrospectively to support the diagnosis. Similarly, Addonizio et al. (1986) proposed that elevated temperature, extrapyramidal symptoms, and a combination of autonomic signs, confusion, and laboratory values could be used to support the diagnosis. These criteria are further codified in DSM-IV (American Psychiatric Association 1994). In criteria proposed by Caroff and colleagues (Caroff et al. 1991; Caroff and Mann 1993), the presence of both muscle rigidity and hyperthermia with temperatures of 38°C or higher are required (Table 1–1). Other associated signs must be present but are considered less critical, less frequent, more variable, difficult to distinguish from pre-NMS findings, or more likely a secondary result of hypermetabolism. In the schema by Caroff and colleagues, diagnostic criteria must specify neuroleptic treatment and underscore that NMS is considered when other neuropsychiatric, systemic, and drug-induced hypermetabolic disorders have been excluded. These criteria emphasize that NMS is a diagnosis of exclusion.

TABLE 1–1.   Diagnostic criteria for neuroleptic malignant syndrome[a]

Treatment with neuroleptics within 7 days of onset
   (2–4 weeks for depot neuroleptics)
Hyperthermia (≥38°C)
Muscle rigidity
Five of the following:
   1. Change in mental status
   2. Tachycardia
   3. Hypertension or hypotension
   4. Tachypnea or hypoxia
   5. Diaphoresis or sialorrhea
   6. Tremor
   7. Incontinence
   8. Creatine phosphokinase elevation or myoglobinuria
   9. Leukocytosis
  10. Metabolic acidosis
Exclusion of other drug-induced, systemic, or neuropsychiatric illnesses

[a]All five criteria required concurrently.
Source. Adapted from Caroff SN, Mann SC, Lazarus A, et al.: "Neuroleptic Malignant Syndrome: Diagnostic Issues." *Psychiatric Annals* 21:130–147, 1991. Used with permission.

Probable or possible NMS cases reported as atypical, in which the full constellation of signs and symptoms (fever, rigidity, autonomic disturbances, and altered mental status) are not present, remain controversial. In such *formes frustes*, either rigidity or hyperthermia did not develop. Whether these instances represent abortive cases of NMS that were detected early, before the full-blown syndrome developed, and then treated promptly or whether these cases fall along a continuum of neuroleptic toxicity of less severity than NMS remains unclear. Addonizio and colleagues (1986) favored the latter explanation in view of their finding that symptoms in these cases sometimes abate without cessation of neuroleptic treatment. On the other hand, Adityanjee et al. (1988) thought that the spectrum concept was an "artifact" based on the "arbitrary" nature by which NMS is defined and diagnosed. However, the heterogeneity and early or partial forms of NMS that have been reported in association with typical antipsychotics are important to note in relation to discussions of whether NMS in association with newer atypical agents is any milder. In fact, a range of severity and completeness of symptoms in NMS cases has been characteristic of the clinical literature.

Ambiguity surrounding the diagnosis of NMS also stems from the fact that some cases reported as NMS were actually unrelated to treatment with antipsychotics. Examples of "nonneuroleptic" malignant syndrome (S. Cohen et al. 1987) include the use of dopamine-depleting agents in a patient with Huntington's disease (Burke et al. 1981) and following withdrawal of dopamine-potentiating drugs in patients with Parkinson's disease, Alzheimer's disease (Rosse and Ciolino 1985), and schizophrenia (Lazarus 1985b). Other cases reported as NMS in the absence of antipsychotics most likely represent instances of serotonin syndrome due to tricyclic antidepressants and monoamine oxidase inhibitors (Brennan et al. 1988; Burch and Downs 1987; S. Cohen et al. 1987; Grant 1984; Ritchie 1983).

Diagnostic criteria for NMS have been derived empirically. There have been few attempts to test the validity, reliability, sensitivity, and specificity of these criteria. Gurrera et al. (1992) compared three sets of criteria in assessing cases diagnosed clinically as NMS and found only modest agreement and consistency. Caroff et al. (2000a) used three sets of criteria to assess reported cases of NMS associated with atypical drugs and observed a range of sensitivity and specificity. Continued investigations designed to test and refine diagnostic criteria and rating instruments for NMS would be worthwhile.

🗿 Clinical Course

The factors involved in the relation between drug exposure and the onset of NMS appear complex. In a review by Caroff and Mann (1988), 16% of the patients developed signs of NMS within 24 hours of initiating neuroleptic treatment, 66% by 1 week, and 96% within 30 days. NMS is less likely to occur after 30 days, but this did happen in 4% of cases.

In some cases, NMS may develop hours after antipsychotic administration (Caroff and Mann 1993). More commonly, NMS evolves over a few days. Early signs may include changes in mental status, extrapyramidal function, and vital signs, as enumerated previously. In most cases, rigidity and mental status changes herald the onset of the syndrome and are secondarily followed by a cascade of systemic signs of hypermetabolism (Velamoor et al. 1994, 1995).

Once neuroleptics are stopped, NMS is self-limited barring complications. Among 65 reported cases involving oral neuroleptics, untreated by dopaminergic agonists or muscle relaxants, the mean recovery time was 9.6 ± 9.1 days (Caroff and Mann 1988). Twenty-three percent recovered in 48 hours, 63% by the end of 1 week, and 97% by the end of 1 month. Other estimates of the mean duration of NMS range from 6.8 to 10.6 days (Deng et al. 1990; Rosebush et al. 1991; M.R. Rosenberg and Green 1989). Patients receiving long-acting depot neuroleptics may have NMS episodes nearly twice as long (Caroff 1980; Deng et al. 1990; Lazarus et al. 1989).

However, symptoms in some cases of NMS persisted apart from treatment with depot drugs. Caroff et al. (2000c) reported on five patients obtained from the database of the Neuroleptic Malignant Syndrome Information Service who developed a residual catatonic and parkinsonian state that persisted over weeks to months after acute hyperthermic symptoms of NMS subsided. In these cases and similar reports in the literature, supportive care and pharmacotherapy were sometimes associated with gradual improvement. However, electroconvulsive therapy (ECT) appeared to be highly effective and rapid in reversing this residual catatonic state that follows NMS in some cases.

Outcome

Despite therapeutic effects, 25 (9.8%) of 256 cases of NMS reported in the literature between 1980 and 1987 ended in death (Caroff and Mann 1988). This represented a decline compared with cases reported before 1980. Shalev et al. (1989) confirmed these findings, showing a decline in mortality from 25% to 11.6% before and after 1984. In Japan, the mortality rate was 28% before 1986 (S. Yamawaki et al. 1988, 1990b). This trend in reduced mortality probably reflects better awareness, early diagnosis, and discontinuation of antipsychotic drugs. It also may reflect the use of specific pharmacological remedies and ECT.

Because of biases in reporting of isolated case reports in the literature, more accurate estimates of mortality have been derived from series of cases studied at individual centers (Lazarus et al. 1989). Such reports support an apparent decline in deaths from nearly 30% to no fatalities in several series (Deng et al. 1990; Keck et al. 1989; Rosebush et al. 1989). Presumably, this decline in case series also reflects greater awareness of the syndrome, early diagnosis, rapid drug discontinuation, institution of supportive care, or use of specific pharmacotherapy and ECT.

In unpublished data, we found that patients reported in the literature who died from NMS were significantly older and developed higher temperatures on average during the NMS episode compared with patients who recovered. In addition, patients who died were significantly more likely to have received depot medications, developed coma, and had evidence of preexisting organic brain pathology. Shalev et al. (1989) found increased mortality associated with prior organic brain syndromes (38.5%) and the development of renal failure (50%). Apart from these data, predictors of outcome are not well established.

Death results from cardiac or respiratory arrest that may occur suddenly or follow cardiac failure, infarction or arrhythmias, aspiration pneumonia, pulmonary emboli, myoglobinuric renal failure, or disseminated intravascular coagulation. Although most patients may be expected to recover from NMS provided the syndrome is recognized, some patients sustain significant morbidity during the course of their illness.

Myoglobinuric renal failure consequent to rhabdomyolysis is one of the more common and more serious complications of NMS and occurs in 16%–25% of cases (Levenson 1985; Shalev and Munitz 1986). Dialysis will be required if renal insufficiency persists, but dialysis will not remove the offending neuroleptic from serum because neuroleptics are highly membrane or protein bound.

It is important to recognize that myoglobinuria has a wide variety of etiologies and may not be as rare as previously thought. The cause of myoglobinuria in NMS is probably multifactorial: immobilization; intramuscular injections; direct drug myotoxicity; muscle necrosis due to severe rigidity, catatonic posturing, or coma; hyperthermia; hypoxia; ischemia; and dehydration. Myoglobinuria may be seen in psychiatric patients with neuroleptic-related conditions other than NMS, for example, in neuroleptic-induced dystonic reactions (Cavanaugh and Finlayson 1984; Ravi et al. 1982), in rapid intramuscular "neuroleptization" (Thase and Shostak 1984), and (rarely) in tardive dyskinesia (Lazarus and Toglia 1985).

Psychiatric patients in particular appear to be at high risk for developing rhabdomyolysis and renal failure (Lazarus 1985c). Psychotropic agents alone may cause rhabdomyolysis, but most case reports involve other factors (Lazarus et al. 1989). Recognizing psychiatric patients who may be at risk for rhabdomyolysis is important because early detection and timely therapy may reduce morbidity and mortality.

Respiratory distress is another frequent complication of NMS. Levenson (1985) observed that ventilator support was necessary for 10 (18.9%) of 53 patients with NMS. Respiratory failure in NMS may be caused by aspiration due to impaired deglutition, infection, shock, pulmonary emboli, acidosis, neuroleptic-induced decreased chest wall compliance, and necrosis of respiratory muscles due to rhabdomyolysis. The normal size and configuration of the cardiac silhouette on chest X ray suggest that pulmonary edema in some cases of NMS may involve noncardiogenic factors (Martin et al. 1985).

Although Delay and Deniker (1968) originally considered respiratory abnormalities an integral part of the NMS symptom complex, other researchers believed that acute respiratory insufficiency in neuroleptic-treated patients constituted a separate entity (Auzepy et al. 1977; Giroud et al. 1978). However, a review (Buffat et al. 1985) of this controversy did not support the distinction. Most patients who developed respiratory insufficiency while taking neuroleptics also showed features common in NMS: extrapyramidal rigidity, hyperthermia, rhabdomyolysis, and a favorable response to dantrolene. It may be that in some patients with NMS, severe respiratory abnormalities predominate; these patients may be predisposed to pulmonary problems on the basis of chronic obstructive pulmonary disease or a preexisting immune deficiency (Buffat et al. 1985).

Persistent neuromuscular abnormalities have been reported in several patients with NMS. Residual muscle stiffness is not uncommon. Rigidity may be severe enough to cause joint subluxation, muscle avulsion, and contractures of the extremities (P.S. Mueller 1985). Other neurological impairments may include permanent dystonia (P.S. Mueller et al. 1983) and polyneuropathy (S.A. Anderson and Weinschenk 1987), resulting in weakness and sensory impairment.

Persistent long-term cognitive sequelae of NMS appear to be rare. Deficits of brain function are related to the severity or complications of the syndrome, particularly hypoxia and extreme or prolonged hyperthermia. However, there have been a few reports of organic amnestic syndromes and extrapyramidal or cerebellar disorders that may persist for weeks, months, or indefinitely (Rosebush and Stewart 1989; Rosebush et al. 1991; van Harten and Kemperman 1991).

Cases of NMS involving the coadministration of lithium and complicated by severe hyperthermia may be more likely to result in cortical and cerebellar damage with cognitive impairment, neuropsychiatric abnormalities, persistent ataxia, dyskinesias, dysarthria, and apraxia (see Chapter 4). The cerebellum has been shown to be particularly sensitive to the effects of lithium salts, even in therapeutic doses (Apte and Langston 1983; Donaldson and Cunningham 1983). In addition, the cerebellum appears to be extremely sensitive to the effects of hyperthermia (Freeman and Dumoff 1944; Malamud et al. 1946).

Autopsy findings in NMS have been nonspecific and variable, depending on complications. Neuropathological findings usually are negative or consistent with the effects of hyperthermia and hypoxia. We found autopsy data reported in 20 fatal cases of NMS (Lazarus et al. 1989). No abnormal CNS findings were seen in 5 cases (P. Henry et al. 1971; H. Itoh et al. 1977; Kinross-Wright 1958; Morris et al. 1980). In 3 cases, no other specific pathology could account for the cause of death (Merriam 1987; Moyes

1973; Straker 1986). Postmortem findings in the remaining cases revealed abnormalities of the brain and viscera generally believed to be the result of hyperthermia, medical complications, or unrelated disorders. For example, "atypical" brain lesions were observed in 3 cases of NMS, probably as a result of the effects of hyperthermia and/or hypoxia rather than as a direct effect of the neuroleptic (Surmont et al. 1984). Likewise, Horn et al. (1988) reported a fatal case of NMS associated with hypothalamic lesions "similar in nature and distribution to those of anoxia-ischemia." This underscores the difficulty in interpreting postmortem findings in NMS because changes may occur secondarily and may not be related directly to underlying pathophysiological mechanisms.

🗟 Differential Diagnosis

The differential diagnosis of NMS encompasses a broad range of disorders presenting with fever, necessitating a thorough medical and neurological evaluation (Table 1–2) (Caroff and Mann 1993; Caroff et al. 1991; Gelenberg 1976). The differential is narrowed by the co-occurrence of the associated features of rigidity, mental status changes, and autonomic dysfunction. Even so, despite careful investigation, the cause of the syndrome in some patients may remain elusive or reflect multiple determinants.

In data obtained from the Neuroleptic Malignant Syndrome Information Service database, the most common syndromes confused with NMS were infections, agitated delirium, and benign extrapyramidal and catatonic symptoms. In a literature review of 48 case reports of NMS, Levinson and Simpson (1986) found 25 cases in which concurrent medical illness could be invoked as the cause of fever. Sewell and Jeste (1992) analyzed 34 patients referred for suspected NMS and found that 10 had acute, serious medical problems, including infections and extrapyramidal symptoms, instead of NMS. They wisely cautioned that when a patient taking neuroleptics develops a febrile syndrome, it is just as important to consider NMS as it is to consider other acute and serious medical illnesses. The differential diagnosis of NMS can be divided into disorders of the CNS and systemic disorders.

Disorders of the Central Nervous System

Infections

Viral encephalitis or postinfectious encephalomyelitis can be difficult to distinguish from NMS, particularly when the presenting signs are behavioral (Caroff et al. 1998b, 2001b). Preexisting viral illness, headaches, meningeal signs, seizures, focal signs, and positive CSF examination or

TABLE 1–2.   Differential diagnosis of neuroleptic malignant syndrome

Primary central nervous system disorders

  Infections (viral encephalitis, human immunodeficiency virus, postinfectious
    encephalomyelitis)

  Tumors

  Cerebrovascular accidents

  Trauma

  Seizures

  Major psychoses (malignant catatonia)

Systemic disorders

  Infections

  Metabolic conditions

  Endocrinopathies (thyroid storm, pheochromocytoma)

  Autoimmune disease (systemic lupus erythematosus)

  Heatstroke

  Toxins (carbon monoxide, phenols, tetanus, strychnine)

  Drugs (salicylates, dopamine inhibitors and antagonists, stimulants,
    psychedelics, monoamine oxidase inhibitors, anesthetics, anticholinergics,
    alcohol or sedative withdrawal)

Source.   Adapted from Caroff SN, Mann SC, Lazarus A, et al.: "Neuroleptic Malignant Syndrome: Diagnostic Issues." *Psychiatric Annals* 21:130–147, 1991. Used with permission.

brain imaging suggest a viral etiology. Several cases of NMS have been re-ported in patients infected with human immunodeficiency virus who also received neuroleptics. In these cases, it may be difficult to distinguish drug effects from viral illness, although discontinuation of neuroleptics may be wise regardless. The predilection of human immunodeficiency virus and other viruses to infect midbrain structures may increase the risk of severe extrapyramidal reactions, including NMS, among infected patients treated with neuroleptics (Caroff and Mann 1993).

Structural Pathology

Anatomical lesions resulting from tumors, abscesses, stroke, or trauma should be evaluated by history, neurological examination, and brain imag-ing (Caroff and Mann 1993). In particular, damage to the anterior cingu-late gyri, mammillary bodies, periventricular nuclei in the hypothalamus, or brain stem areas may produce akinetic mutism resembling NMS, possi-bly caused by damage to dopamine tracts passing through these regions (Mann et al. 1991). In contrast to these cases with diagnosable brain le-sions, brain imaging and postmortem examination of NMS patients have found no consistent or specific pattern of brain pathology.

Seizures

Rarely, cases of nonconvulsive status epilepticus with stupor may resemble NMS. Confusion may result from the fact that neuroleptics may lower the seizure threshold, and fever and CPK elevations may occur after convulsive activity. However, seizures are not commonly observed in NMS and should prompt a search for metabolic or structural causes.

Major Psychoses (Malignant Catatonia)

The potentially lethal progression of catatonic and manic states in psychotic disorders has been well described for more than a century (Chapter 5). In these cases, unchecked hyperactivity can lead to exhaustion, stupor, hyperthermia, and death (Mann et al. 1986; Stauder 1934). Sometimes, a uniformly stuporous course with rigidity indistinguishable from that of NMS may occur. Although the incidence of malignant catatonia may have decreased, it must be considered when hyperthermia develops in an agitated and untreated psychotic patient. Differentiation from NMS in a neuroleptic-treated stuporous patient is more difficult. In either case, however, discontinuation of neuroleptics may be indicated; in most NMS cases, symptoms should resolve in 1–2 weeks, and in malignant catatonia, neuroleptics appear to be ineffective and may further compromise thermoregulation. In fact, open trials suggest that ECT is the treatment of choice in malignant catatonia (Mann et al. 1990).

Systemic Disorders

Extrapyramidal Symptoms With Fever

Intercurrent fever caused by infections or metabolic disorders may develop in patients who also have parkinsonism or catatonia related to neuroleptic treatment (Caroff and Mann 1993; Caroff et al. 1991; Levinson and Simpson 1986; Stoudemire and Luther 1984). The importance of excluding common causes of fever in these patients before diagnosing NMS is critical. Negative medical, laboratory, and postmortem evidence of infectious processes is the rule in most NMS cases. Distinguishing between benign drug-induced extrapyramidal symptoms accompanied by concomitant medical illness causing fever and NMS can be challenging.

Myonecrosis and CPK elevations also have occurred in association with neuroleptic administration and extrapyramidal symptoms, apart from hyperthermia and other signs of NMS. The mechanism of this effect has never been adequately resolved. Whether this is independent of NMS or reflects the same mechanisms as a marker or risk factor remains to be determined (Gurrera and Romero 1993; Manor et al. 1998; Meltzer et al. 1996).

Hormonal Disorders

Extreme hyperthermia may be observed in thyrotoxicosis and pheochromocytoma (Caroff and Mann 1993; Caroff et al. 1991). Hyperthyroid patients may manifest tremor, tachycardia, diaphoresis, and elevated temperatures reminiscent of prodromal signs of NMS. Thyroid storm has been mistaken for MH during surgery, although unlike in MH and NMS, muscle rigidity and rhabdomyolysis are not usually observed. Diagnosis is further complicated by the fact that hyperthyroidism may predispose patients to develop severe rigidity while taking neuroleptics, and neuroleptics may precipitate thyroid storm.

In patients with pheochromocytoma, an acute crisis that may be precipitated by psychotropic drugs may resemble NMS. Although rigidity is not known to occur, significant rhabdomyolysis contributing to renal failure has been reported. It may be difficult to diagnose pheochromocytoma on the basis of plasma or urinary catecholamines because these values may be strikingly elevated in NMS as well (Caroff and Mann 1988, 1988; Caroff et al. 1991).

Autoimmune Disorders

Systemic lupus erythematosus or mixed connective tissue diseases may present with fever, meningitis, and mental status and movement disorders and may be confused with NMS if neuroleptics are prescribed for behavioral manifestations or steroid psychosis (Caroff and Mann 1993; Caroff et al. 1991).

Heatstroke

During hot weather, agitated patients are at risk for exertional heatstroke characterized by sweating, hypotension, high temperatures, acidosis, and rhabdomyolysis, which may progress to renal failure, disseminated intravascular coagulation, and death (Caroff and Mann 1993; Caroff et al. 2000b; Lazarus et al. 1989; Mann and Boger 1978). Administration of neuroleptics increases the risk of heatstroke, although most cases of heatstroke associated with neuroleptics resemble classic rather than exertional heatstroke (see Chapter 2). The classic form is not related to exertion and is characterized by anhidrosis and respiratory alkalosis. Unlike NMS, neither form of heatstroke is typically associated with muscle rigidity. Although clinicians should be aware that neuroleptics increase the risk of heatstroke in hot weather, NMS may occur in patients at rest independent of ambient temperature. Coadministration of anticholinergic drugs significantly compounds the impairment of thermoregulation. In fact, heatstroke is more often associated with low-potency neuroleptics, which possess anticholinergic properties, in contrast to NMS, which is associated more often with high-potency drugs.

Toxins and Drugs

Hyperthermia has been reported with occupational exposure to phenolic compounds and, with muscle rigidity, has also followed carbon monoxide poisoning and L-asparaginase toxicity (Caroff and Mann 1993; Caroff et al. 1991). Other toxins to consider are fluoride and iron salts, strychnine, methylphenyltetrahydropyridine (MPTP), and tetanus or staphylococcal toxins.

Hyperthermia and NMS-like states also have been described in association with drugs of abuse and with prescription drugs other than neuroleptics or antipsychotics (Chapter 4). Stimulants, such as cocaine and forms of amphetamines, produce hyperthermia as a result of agitation, seizures, or muscle rigidity compounded by impaired heat loss due to vasoconstriction. Hyperthermia is a well-known complication and cause of death from abuse of these drugs. Use of 3,4-methylenedioxymethamphetamine (MDMA) or "Ecstasy" has been implicated in hyperthermic states and may cause the serotonin syndrome (Chapters 3 and 4). Psychedelic drugs also cause hyperthermia (Chapter 4). Phencyclidine intoxication may result in rigidity and rhabdomyolysis in addition to temperature elevations.

Withdrawal from alcohol or sedative-hypnotics may be confused with NMS because of mental status changes, autonomic dysfunction, and elevated temperatures in both conditions (Caroff and Mann 1993). Rigidity is not associated with delirium tremens, although rhabdomyolysis may be found in alcoholic patients. The diagnosis may be obscured if neuroleptics are administered during withdrawal. Withdrawal also may increase the risk of NMS. In view of this, as well as their tendency to lower the seizure threshold, neuroleptics should be used cautiously in these patients.

Hyperthermia also has been reported in association with several classes of prescription drugs (Caroff and Mann 1993; Lazarus et al. 1989). By uncoupling oxidative phosphorylation, salicylates may induce hypermetabolism and hyperthermia after acute intoxication or chronic use. Hyperthermia associated with anticholinergic toxicity is also a consideration in the diagnosis of NMS but may be distinguished by the absence of rigidity, presence of atropinic signs, and response to physostigmine.

A great deal of interest was generated by the overlapping clinical features of NMS and MH (Caroff et al. 1994a, 1994b, 2001c; Lazarus et al. 1989). MH is another drug-induced hypermetabolic syndrome that is associated with the administration of anesthetic gases and succinylcholine during anesthesia. Although the clinical features of NMS and MH may be indistinguishable, the preponderance of evidence suggests that the mechanisms underlying these disorders are distinct and that the potential for susceptibility or cross-reactivity to both syndromes in the same patient is unproven.

On a clinical basis, MH is considered in the differential diagnosis of NMS only in the perioperative setting where both anesthetics and neuroleptics may be used. In a literature review of NMS cases occurring in the perioperative setting, Caroff et al. (2001c) found several features that may help in diagnosis. First, NMS does not appear to occur intraoperatively, in contrast to MH, because anesthetics and peripheral skeletal muscle relaxants probably inhibit or mask the centrally driven features of NMS. By contrast, MH is triggered intraoperatively, and postanesthesia and "awake" episodes are more controversial. Although both disorders may respond to dantrolene, which acts on the intracellular concentrations of calcium, only NMS responds to nondepolarizing muscle relaxants, centrally active drugs, and ECT.

Centrally active medications other than antipsychotics also may produce an NMS-like picture. Antidopaminergic drugs, such as metoclopramide, amoxapine, prochlorperazine, tetrabenazine, and reserpine, reduce dopamine activity and have produced hyperthermia. Similarly, withdrawal of dopaminergic agonists, such as levodopa, amantadine, and others used in the treatment of parkinsonian states, has resulted in an NMS-like picture (Chapter 4). In fact, cases of hyperthermia have even been reported in patients with Parkinson's disease during "off" or "freezing" episodes as a result of the "wearing-off" effect of levodopa treatment. These nonneuroleptic drug reactions share the common element of acute reduction in brain dopamine activity, thereby confirming the causal connection between the dopamine antagonist properties of neuroleptics and the clinical signs of NMS.

Lithium by itself is an unlikely cause of rigidity or hyperthermia, although lithium intoxication is associated with a toxic encephalopathy (Chapter 4). Some clinical evidence suggests that lithium combined with neuroleptics may increase the risk of extrapyramidal reactions or NMS. Moreover, the presence of lithium during an NMS episode may predispose the patient to develop lithium intoxication, secondary to dehydration and renal failure, with resulting increased risk of encephalopathy and brain damage.

Baclofen, administered by mouth or by direct CSF infusion, has been used to treat spasticity. Several cases of NMS-like reactions have been associated with baclofen withdrawal or failure of baclofen pumps (Chapter 4).

Finally, there has been a proliferation of case reports and reviews of the serotonin syndrome and its relation to NMS (Chapter 3). The serotonin syndrome consists of a spectrum of behavioral, autonomic, and neuromuscular symptoms associated with the use of serotoninergic drugs (Keck and Arnold 2000; P.J. Mason et al. 2000). With the increase in the development of these drugs in the treatment of depression, anxiety, and migraines, the incidence of this disorder has undoubtedly increased.

In most instances, the serotonin syndrome differs from NMS in presentation, course, and prognosis. Serotonin syndrome results most often from the use of drug combinations or overdose. Serotonin syndrome usually develops rapidly, within 24 hours, and subsides rapidly if diagnosed, medications are stopped, and treatment is administered. Some evidence suggests that serotonin antagonists, such as cyproheptadine, may facilitate recovery as opposed to dopaminergic and other agents in NMS.

In most cases, serotonin syndrome presents as an agitated delirium with confusion, restlessness, myoclonus, and tachycardia as typical features. Although this presentation is easily distinguished from NMS, serotonin syndrome occasionally can progress to a fulminant hypermetabolic state identical to NMS and has responded to dantrolene in some instances. This extreme form of serotonin syndrome is associated primarily with monoamine oxidase inhibitors.

🐚 Treatment

The basis of treatment of NMS remains reduction of risk factors; early recognition; cessation of neuroleptic medication; and institution of intensive medical care focusing on fluid replacement, reduction of temperature, and support of cardiac, respiratory, and renal functions (Caroff and Mann 1993; J.M. Davis et al. 2000). Careful monitoring for complications, particularly cardiorespiratory failure, aspiration pneumonia, thromboembolism, and renal failure, is essential. The favorable outcomes obtained in prospective studies provide support for this fundamental approach (Deng et al. 1990; Gelenberg et al. 1989; Keck et al. 1991; Rosebush and Stewart 1989).

The development of elevated body temperature in a patient taking neuroleptics should always be a cause for concern and prompt medical attention. When hyperthermia is accompanied by rigidity, deterioration in neurological status, and autonomic instability, NMS must be considered. Hyperthermia in combination with neurological changes obligates the clinician to consider stopping neuroleptic drugs until a specific etiology is discovered or until symptoms resolve.

Discontinuation of neuroleptics is significantly correlated with recovery from NMS (Addonizio et al. 1987). In 65 reported cases involving oral neuroleptics (and not treated with dantrolene or dopaminergic agonists), the mean±SD recovery time after drug discontinuation was 9.6±9.1 days

(Caroff and Mann 1988); 23% recovered in 48 hours, 63% by 1 week, 82% by 2 weeks, and 97% by the end of a month.

Lithium, antidepressants, and medications with potent anticholinergic activity should be discontinued. Whether these drugs offer some prophylactic advantage or, on the contrary, predispose to or complicate NMS is unclear. It may be hazardous to continue lithium in a dehydrated, hyperthermic patient. Similarly, drugs with potent anticholinergic properties may inhibit sweating and further impair heat loss. However, dopamine agonist medication (e.g., amantadine, levodopa) should not be discontinued. Abrupt withdrawal of dopamine agonists may precipitate or exacerbate symptoms in NMS (D.M. Simpson and Davis 1984). Their continued use during an acute episode of NMS may, theoretically, decrease the severity of symptoms.

Medical Management

Supportive medical and nursing management of vital functions and treatment of complications are essential (J.M. Davis et al. 2000). Extreme hyperthermia constitutes a medical emergency; it should be treated vigorously because it is predictive of morbidity and mortality. High temperatures combined with hypoxia are significant risk factors for brain damage. Patients are quickly dehydrated by poor intake and diaphoresis so that intravenous fluids are critical in preventing hypovolemia, impaired heat loss, circulatory collapse, and renal failure. Acid–base abnormalities should be monitored and corrected. Respiratory failure is common and may occur precipitously, requiring intubation and ventilatory support. This may occur secondary to increased respiratory demand, coupled with constricting rigidity of chest wall musculature. Aspiration is a frequent complication. Muscle hypermetabolism and rigidity, in the face of temperature elevations, hypovolemia, and ischemia, may lead to muscle necrosis and rhabdomyolysis, measured by elevated serum muscle enzymes and myoglobinuria (J.M. Davis et al. 2000). Although usually in the range of a few thousand, CPK elevations may be pronounced and result in myoglobinuric renal failure that requires dialysis. Antipsychotic medications, however, are not dialyzable. Muscle rigidity and necrosis, hyperthermia, and ischemia also trigger thromboembolic phenomena, resulting in venous thrombosis, pulmonary emboli, and disseminated intravascular coagulation. Subcutaneous heparin may be indicated as prophylaxis.

Specific Treatment

Because NMS in most instances may be a self-limited disorder if recognized early, discontinuation of triggering drugs and medical or supportive therapy are paramount and may be sufficient for recovery. Beyond support-ive therapy, the role of specific pharmacological agents and ECT in the treatment of NMS is unresolved. Controlled, prospective data comparing specific treatments with supportive care are lacking; most reports rely on retrospective, anecdotal, and clinical reports or small case series. Neverthe-less, impressive theoretical reasons and data from meta-analyses of the clin-ical literature suggest the potential value of these treatments, which were reviewed previously (J.M. Davis et al. 2000) and are summarized next.

Benzodiazepines

Viewing NMS as a form of catatonia, several investigators have proposed using benzodiazepines as a first-line treatment (J.M. Davis et al. 2000; Fink 1996; Francis et al. 2000; Fricchione et al. 1997). Indeed, benzodiazepines have been effective in cases of NMS (Francis et al. 2000; Fricchione et al. 2000), particularly those with milder symptomatology. In some cases, ben-zodiazepines were effective when other medications failed (Miyaoka et al. 1997). In a report by Francis et al. (2000), rigidity and fever abated in 24–48 hours, whereas other secondary features of NMS were relieved within 64 hours without adverse effects.

Still, benzodiazepines have not been uniformly effective in all cases and, at times, have had only a transitory effect. Furthermore, they did not prevent NMS from developing in controlled studies of risk factors (Caroff and Mann 1993; Keck et al. 1989; Shalev and Munitz 1986). A trial of 1–2 mg of lorazepam intramuscularly or intravenously may be indicated in cases of NMS, with monitoring of respiratory status. For patients who respond, a switch to oral doses of lorazepam can maintain the therapeutic effect.

Dopamine Agonists

Substantial evidence suggests that NMS results from an acute reduction in dopaminergic function in the brain, such that dopaminergic agonists may reverse this deficit and facilitate resolution of the syndrome (J.M. Davis et al. 2000; Mann et al. 2000). There is clear evidence for the effectiveness of amantadine in NMS. In a previous analysis, amantadine was used in 34 cases and as the sole treatment in 19 (Sakkas et al. 1991). More than half of the clinicians reported amantadine to be beneficial in recovery, and 63% reported improvement when it was used as monotherapy. Only one death was reported among patients treated with amantadine. This finding was statistically significant ($P=0.03$) among cases in which amantadine was used in combination but only a strong trend when amantadine was used alone because of the smaller number of cases. NMS clearly worsened when amantadine was discontinued in six patients. Although we list amantadine under dopaminergic agents, it may be acting as an N-methyl-D-aspartate receptor antagonist in addition to promoting the release of endogenous dopamine. The dose is usually 200–400 mg/day given orally in divided doses. Amantadine may exacerbate psychotic symptoms but is usually well tolerated.

One hundred patients who received bromocriptine were also analyzed (Sakkas et al. 1991); bromocriptine was used as monotherapy for half of the patients. Clinicians reported a beneficial effect in 88% of the patients when bromocriptine was used in combination and in 94% of the patients when bromocriptine was used alone. The mortality rate was reduced by 50% in patients who were given bromocriptine compared with those given supportive treatment alone, whether used as monotherapy ($P=0.04$) or in combination ($P=0.02$). NMS symptomatology worsened in 10 patients following discontinuation of bromocriptine, 3 of whom received it as monotherapy. In agreement with these findings, M.R. Rosenberg and Green (1989) analyzed 67 published cases of NMS and reported that bromocriptine significantly shortened the time to clinical response (1.03 ± 0.55 days) compared with supportive treatment alone (6.80 ± 2.68 days). In a survey of 492 cases of NMS in Japan, S. Yamawaki et al. (1990b) reported that 27 (81.8%) of 33 patients treated with bromocriptine showed a positive response.

In our opinion, evidence of clinical efficacy supports the use of bromocriptine in NMS. The starting dose of bromocriptine is 2.5 mg orally given two or three times a day, increased to a total daily dose of 45 mg if necessary. Bromocriptine can worsen psychosis and contribute to changes in blood pressure. Vomiting can occur with risk of aspiration in obtunded patients.

Levodopa has been used in only a limited number of cases, and clinicians thought it was effective in approximately half of the cases (Sakkas et al. 1991). It was used as monotherapy in only 12 patients. The data are insufficient for a statistical analysis. However, some dramatic improvements occurred with levodopa, even after failure to respond to dantrolene (Nisijima et al. 1997). Additional dopaminergic-enhancing medications introduced for the treatment of Parkinson's disease, including tolcapone, pramipexole, ropinirole, and pergolide, deserve further study. These medications may be beneficial in treating NMS, but, conversely, abrupt withdrawal may result in the development of NMS-like syndromes.

Anticholinergic Medications

There have been a few cases of NMS in which anticholinergic medications were believed to be beneficial (J.M. Davis et al. 2000). However, for patients with high temperatures, for whom sweating is an essential means of reducing temperature, anticholinergic blockade can seriously compromise effective thermoregulation. Anticholinergic medications are not recommended for treating NMS or other hyperthermic conditions. NMS has been reported following abrupt withdrawal of anticholinergic or other antiparkinsonian medications; therefore, these medications should be tapered gradually.

Dantrolene

Temperature elevations in NMS probably result from antipsychotic-induced impairment of central heat loss mechanisms in combination with excess heat production secondary to peripheral hypermetabolism and rigidity of skeletal muscle. Muscle relaxants may be helpful in reducing the generation of heat in muscle, the body's primary source of internal heat.

Dantrolene, which inhibits contraction and heat production in muscle, has been successfully used in treating MH during anesthesia as well as other hypermetabolic disorders. Its action is misunderstood; it is not specific for MH but may be effective in reducing endogenous heat generation regardless of etiology. Cases of NMS with extreme temperature elevations may benefit from treatment with dantrolene. The exact temperature elevation necessary for dantrolene is a matter of judgment. However, patients who have temperatures in excess of 40°C, with severe rigidity and rhabdomyolysis, are probably the best candidates for dantrolene. Conversely, mild cases with catatonia and low-grade temperatures may not benefit at all.

Dantrolene can be combined safely with benzodiazepines or dopamine agonists but has been associated with cardiovascular collapse if administered in combination with calcium-channel blockers. Side effects of dantrolene may include impairment of respiratory or hepatic function, which should be monitored.

In a previous report, dantrolene had been used in more than 100 cases and was the only medication used in 50% of these (Sakkas et al. 1991). Clinicians reported that 81% of the patients were helped by dantrolene. Clinical improvement and muscle relaxation sometimes started within minutes of administration, and beneficial effects were readily apparent in the next few hours (A. Henderson and Longdon 1991). Relapse on discontinuation of dantrolene occurred in eight patients, including two patients in whom dantrolene was the only medication used, thereby providing important evidence for the efficacy of the medication. In addition, dantrolene significantly reduced mortality by half compared with supportive care, whether used alone ($P=0.04$) or in combination ($P=0.01$). M.R. Rosenberg and Green (1989) found that dantrolene reduced the response time to

1.72±1.15 days when compared with supportive care alone (6.80±2.68 days). S. Yamawaki et al. (1990b) reported a positive response to dantrolene in 105 (74.5%) of 141 patients with NMS who received it. In a later study of NMS, S. Yamawaki et al. (1993) reported that dantrolene resulted in moderate improvement or better in 15 (55.6%) of 27 cases and slight improvement or better in 21 (77.8%) of 27 cases; only 1 patient died (3.7%). Tsutsumi et al. (1998) reported that dantrolene was primarily effective in reducing muscle rigidity and less effective in treating disturbances of consciousness in 21 patients with NMS.

For MH of anesthesia, dantrolene is initially given as 1.0–2.5 mg/kg intravenously. If acidosis, rigidity, and temperature resolve, then 1.0 mg/kg every 6 hours is administered for 48 hours. If the patient is not acidotic and appears weak, then 1.0 mg/kg can be given every 12 hours. Tsutsumi et al. (1998) concluded that for NMS, the standard intravenous dose and period of administration of dantrolene should be 1 mg/kg/day and 8 days, respectively. Dantrolene can be continued in oral form for 1 week or more following response to intravenous therapy.

In contrast to the studies mentioned previously in this chapter, Rosebush et al. (1991) reported that patients treated with bromocriptine ($n=2$), dantrolene ($n=2$), or both ($n=4$) had a longer course and more sequelae than did patients treated with supportive care alone, although patients were not randomized, and patients treated with medications had a higher incidence of preexisting serious medical illnesses. Shalev and Munitz (1986) found significantly reduced mortality in reported cases of NMS treated with dopamine agonists or dantrolene but noted that this effect was diminished when controlled for the overall reduction in mortality among cases of NMS published after 1984.

ECT

All of the pharmacological agents mentioned are generally effective within the first few days of NMS (J.M. Davis et al. 2000). If, despite adequate dosing, a response has not been obtained after a few days, a delayed response is unlikely, and ECT becomes an important consideration. ECT has been highly effective in catatonia and also has been reported to be effective in the treatment of Parkinson's disease (Kellner et al. 1994), perhaps underscoring the effect of ECT in increasing dopamine synthesis and release. Not surprisingly, ECT also has been effective in treating NMS during the acute stage (J.M. Davis et al. 1991; Mann et al. 1990) and in the event of the development of a prolonged, residual catatonic or parkinsonian state following NMS (Caroff et al. 2000c).

J.M. Davis et al. (1991) reported that the mortality rate of patients treated with ECT was 10.3% compared with 9.7% for patients treated with medications and 21% for patients treated with supportive care alone. They found that patients who did not respond to ECT had continued to take antipsychotics. Mann et al. (1990) reported ECT as effective in 23 (85.2%) of 27 cases of NMS published in the literature. Scheftner and Shulman (1992) reported that the mean time to clinical response after the first ECT treatment was 1.46±2.38 days in NMS episodes, with most patients responding within 72 hours. Nisijima and Ishiguro (1999) reported that the mean time to complete resolution was 6.0 days in five patients with NMS and psychotic symptoms who received ECT. Similarly, Trollor and Sachdev (1999) proposed ECT as the preferred treatment in severe NMS, or when psychotic depression, catatonia, or malignant catatonia is involved, based on a review of 54 case reports. They found that ECT resulted in complete recovery in 63% of the patients and in partial recovery in another 28%.

ECT offers the unique advantage of treating not only NMS but also the underlying psychosis. Although Sachdev et al. (1997) reported that prior ECT appeared to be a risk factor for NMS, this more likely reflects the fact that patients with ECT-responsive states experienced in their past, notably catatonia, are also susceptible to NMS. Patients with NMS are not considered to be at risk for MH during ECT; however, clinicians should be aware that succinylcholine can cause hyperkalemia and arrhythmias in patients with rhabdomyolysis, which may explain instances of cardiac complications in patients with NMS who receive ECT. Other muscle relaxants should be considered for patients with significant rhabdomyolysis who are at risk.

Treatment Summary

In conclusion, the principal management of NMS remains attempts at prevention through the conservative use of antipsychotics, reduction of risk factors, and early diagnosis with prompt discontinuation of triggering medications. In view of the heterogeneity of cases diagnosed as NMS, differing theoretical opinions, and the lack of prospective, controlled trials and standardized dosing, it may be premature to exclusively recommend supportive care, ECT, or one pharmacological intervention over others for all cases of NMS. Anecdotal reports in the literature, which are used to support specific treatments, are often confounded by the fact that some cases may represent early cases of benign extrapyramidal symptoms that would not progress to NMS, whereas other severe cases of NMS entail a worse prognosis regardless of specific treatment. We believe that specific treatment of NMS should be individualized and based empirically on the character, duration, and severity of clinical signs and symptoms (Caroff et al. 1998a; J.M. Davis et al. 2000; Woodbury and Woodbury 1992). In many cases, especially with mild or early signs, supportive care with close monitoring for progression of symptoms or the development of complications is probably sufficient until recovery occurs (Rosebush et al. 1991). Anticholinergic medications are essential for afebrile patients experiencing antipsychotic-induced parkinsonian symptoms but complicate the management of hyperthermic patients and should be tapered off once fever develops. Benzodiazepines and amantadine are effective in treating neuroleptic-induced catatonia, which may precede NMS in some cases. Benzodiazepines are useful in controlling agitation and in reversing catatonic and other symptoms of NMS. They are easy to administer and could be tried in most cases.

Trials of bromocriptine, amantadine, or other dopamine agonists may be a reasonable next step for patients with at least moderate symptoms of NMS (e.g., rigidity and temperatures of 38.3°C to 40.0°C). Dantrolene appears to be beneficial primarily in cases involving significant muscle rigidity, hypermetabolism, and hyperthermia, with temperatures exceeding 40°C. All of these medications generally show an effect during the first few days of treatment and may be unlikely to show a delayed response thereafter.

In contrast, ECT may be effective even late in the course, after other interventions have failed (Scheftner and Shulman 1992). ECT may be preferred if idiopathic malignant catatonia cannot be excluded, if NMS is refractory to supportive care and pharmacotherapy, in patients with prominent catatonic features who are not responsive to benzodiazepines, and in patients who have a residual post-NMS catatonic state or remain psychotic after NMS has resolved. Further clarification of the best treatment approach with specific interventions requires additional data from future studies.

Rechallenge and Recurrence

After recovery from NMS, patients may require treatment with neuroleptics for the reemergence of psychotic disorders (Caroff and Mann 1993). In reviewing the literature, Shalev and Munitz (1986) found recurrence of NMS with two fatalities in 50% of 24 patients rechallenged with neuroleptics. They recommended use of low-potency drugs because the recurrence rate declined to 10% in cases treated with thioridazine. Similarly, Caroff and Mann (1988) reported recurrence in 14 (29.8%) of 47 patients, which declined to 15% when low-potency drugs were used. Gelenberg et al. (1989) treated six patients who had NMS previously, four of whom received thioridazine without recurrence, although one patient developed elevated temperature and CPK elevations when briefly treated with the more potent drug loxapine. In a review of reports of NMS associated with atypical antipsychotics, Caroff et al. (2000a) found that clozapine, risperidone, olanzapine, and quetiapine were associated with recurrence of definite or possible symptoms of NMS when used in patients who had a previous episode of NMS.

Wells et al. (1988) reported that recurrence of symptoms doubled when neuroleptics were reintroduced within 5 days of recovery. Susman and Addonizio (1988) found that 15 (42.9%) of 35 patients experienced recurrence. They noted that retreatment before 2 weeks elapsed after recovery increased the risk of recurrence. However, three of their own patients developed recurrences as late as 7–24 months after the initial episode. Rosebush et al. (1989) reported neuroleptic rechallenge in 15 patients over a 6-year period and found that 13 (86.7%) were eventually able to take neuroleptics safely. However, on initial rechallenge, 5 (33.3%) of the 15 patients experienced partial or complete recurrence of NMS. Rosebush et al. (1989) also found a significant effect of time from recovery but failed to show a clear relation between recurrence and drug potency or dosage. However, the numbers of patients in these studies may be too small to separate parameters of drug use from the time of administration and other variables.

Pope et al. (1991) found only one possible recurrent episode of NMS during 16 years of subsequent neuroleptic exposure and 71 years of previous exposure in 20 patients studied after a single episode of NMS and concluded that individual predisposition contributed only modestly to the risk of recurrence compared with state-related cofactors that remain unclear. However, compared with the risk of NMS in all neuroleptic-treated patients (0.2% or less), the risk of recurrence, about 30% in some studies, suggests that certain patients may be inherently susceptible.

Most patients can be safely treated with neuroleptics after NMS, provided certain guidelines to reduce the risk are followed (Caroff and Mann 1993). Previous episodes of NMS should be thoroughly reviewed for accuracy of diagnosis. After recovery, the indications for treatment with neuroleptics should be assessed and documented. Alternative treatments should be considered. Informed consent from the patient and family is advisable. Potential risk factors, such as dehydration, agitation, and concomitant medical illness, should be minimized. At least 2 weeks should elapse after complete recovery from NMS before neuroleptics are administered. Although data on neuroleptic potency are inconclusive, gradual titration of low doses of low-potency or atypical drugs may be safest. Patients should be monitored in the hospital for incipient signs of NMS. Some clinicians have advocated prophylactic treatment with dantrolene or dopamine agonists, although there is no evidence that this offers advantages over conservative management.

🗿 Pathogenesis

Dopamine

Several hypotheses have been proposed to explain the pathogenesis of NMS. The most compelling evidence supports the occurrence of central dopamine hypoactivity as the principal factor in the development of NMS (Caroff and Mann 1993; Mann et al. 1991, 2000). All neuroleptic or antipsychotic drugs implicated in NMS share the property of D_2 dopamine receptor antagonism. Although it has been difficult to conclusively show a correlation between NMS and drug dosage or potency, evidence from studies of incidence (Gelenberg et al. 1989; Keck et al. 1991) rate, route of drug administration (Keck et al. 1989), and recurrences (Caroff and Mann 1988) supports a positive correlation. Other drugs such as metoclopramide and amoxapine, which are dopamine antagonists but not used as antipsychotics, have been known to cause NMS. Most important, patients treated with dopamine agonists for idiopathic Parkinson's disease have developed NMS-like states when drugs were withdrawn or lost effectiveness. In addition, dopamine agonists appear to be effective in treating NMS and may contribute to recrudescence of symptoms if withdrawn prematurely (Sakkas et al. 1991).

Furthermore, Spivak et al. (2000) found a significant decrease in dopamine concentrations in plasma from NMS patients. Suzuki et al. (2001) and Ram et al. (1995) reported abnormalities in the D_2 dopamine receptor gene.

In reviewing neuroanatomical correlates of NMS, Mann et al. (1991, 2000) analyzed reports of NMS-like disorders in patients with lesions involving the anterior cingulate gyri, mammillary bodies, periventricular nuclei in the hypothalamus, or brain stem areas, perhaps as a result of interruption of dopaminergic tracts passing through these regions. Postmortem findings have not revealed specific or consistent patterns of neuropathology in the brains of NMS patients. Autopsy findings have included cerebellar degeneration (Kish et al. 1990; S. Lee et al. 1989), necrosis of hypothalamic nuclei, cell loss in the nucleus basalis (in lethal catatonia treated with neuroleptics) (Kish et al. 1990), ischemic/anoxic changes (Becker et al. 1992; Shalev et al. 1989), or no changes at all (E.M. Jones and Dawson 1989).

Kish et al. (1990) found normal levels of hypothalamic and striatal dopamine and D_2 dopamine receptor binding in the brains of three patients with fatal hyperthermic syndromes but noted that the reduced level of homovanillic acid (HVA) in two of the patients suggested reduced capacity of the dopamine system to compensate for stress or neuroleptic-induced receptor blockade. In this study, a profound reduction in choline acetyl-transferase in the cortex and limbic system was found, in addition to marked reduction in hypothalamic noradrenaline, prompting Kish et al. (1990) to speculate that striatal dopamine dysfunction and cholinergic hypoactivity predispose to NMS, whereas noradrenaline depletion may result secondarily from stress and hyperthermia. Gertz and Schmidt (1991) suggested dopamine hypoactivity in one case of NMS in which they noted a striking loss of melanin as a breakdown product in the substantia nigra. Finally, DeReuck et al. (1991) performed positron emission tomography in three NMS patients and found increased metabolism in the striatum, cerebellum, and occipital cortex in two patients, which they interpreted as implicating neurotransmitter systems in addition to dopamine in the pathogenesis of the syndrome. Jauss et al. (1996) reported virtually complete blockade of D_2 dopamine receptors in a patient with NMS who was studied with single photon emission computed tomography scans.

Further evidence for hypodopaminergia in NMS derives from investigations of neurotransmitter metabolites in the CSF. Findings from studies of levels of dopamine and its major metabolite HVA have been inconsistent in single case reports (Lazarus et al. 1989). However, Nisijima and Ishiguro (1990, 1995a) found consistent evidence of significantly reduced HVA levels in patients compared with control subjects, both during and after recovery from NMS. These findings were further strengthened by a recent report showing significant reductions in CSF levels of HVA in patients with Parkinson's disease who developed NMS compared with control subjects (Ueda et al. 1999).

Collectively, these findings suggest that patients susceptible to developing NMS may have baseline central hypodopaminergia as a trait vulnerability for the disorder (Mann et al. 2000) that is exacerbated following further stress and pharmacologically induced reductions in dopamine activity. Based on current understanding of basal ganglia–thalamocortical circuits, Mann et al. (2000) further reviewed how these reductions could account for the major manifestations of the disorder. Muscular rigidity may result from impaired dopaminergic transmission in the motor circuit, whereas decreased dopaminergic input to the anterior cingulate-medial orbitofrontal circuit could account for akinetic mutism. In addition, blockade of the lateral orbitofrontal circuit might underlie other selected catatonic features of NMS. Furthermore, dopaminergic antagonism in the anterior cingulate-medial orbitofrontal circuit may also participate in causing hyperthermia and autonomic dysfunction in concert with dopmaine receptor blockade involving diencephalospinal dopamine pathways, hypothalamic dopamine neurons, and peripheral dopamine receptors (see Chaper 5).

Other Neurotransmitter Systems

Although the direct and indirect evidence for central hypodopaminergia appears compelling, alternative factors have been proposed as contributing to the development of NMS in a particular patient. Weller and Kornhuber (1992a) and Kornhuber et al. (1993) have emphasized that NMS may reflect relative glutaminergic transmission excess as a consequence of dopaminergic blockade.

Rosebush and Mazurek (1991) and J. W. Y. Lee (1998) reported the association between low serum iron levels as a marker or risk factor for NMS. They speculated that low iron concentration levels in NMS may contribute to triggering an episode based on evidence that iron may play an integral role in the normal functioning of central D_2 dopamine receptors.

Based on pharmacological responses in patients and postmortem and CSF studies, several authors have proposed the potential involvement of norepinephrine, γ-aminobutyric acid (GABA), serotonin, and opioid neurotransmitters in the triggering of NMS (Lazarus et al. 1989; Mann et al. 1991, 2000).

In an extensive review of competing theories, Gurrera (1999) postulated that drug-induced disruption of central inhibitory inputs leads to dysregulation and hyperactivity of the sympathetic nervous system. This results in excessive stimulation of thermoeffector end organs manifested by increased muscle tone and metabolism, increased mitochondrial thermogenesis, ineffective heat dissipation, fluctuations in vasomotor tone, granulocytosis, and urinary incontinence.

Skeletal Muscle Pathology

Apart from central dopaminergic hypoactivity, effects of other neurotransmitters, and sympathetic nervous system dysfunction, NMS has prompted research into neuromuscular mechanisms underlying hyperthermia (Caroff et al. 1994a, 1994b, 2001c; Lazarus et al. 1989). These investigations have been stimulated in part because of the clinical similarities between NMS and MH of anesthesia.

However, significant differences exist between the syndromes (Keck et al. 1995). For example, NMS can occur in milder variants, appearing primarily as a catatonic or extrapyramidal disorder. NMS may respond to centrally active drugs and ECT. NMS is more common than MH; unlike MH, it develops gradually and is of longer duration than MH. These distinguishing features reflect the different pathogenetic mechanisms underlying the two syndromes; NMS is considered a manifestation of hypodopaminergia in the brain (Mann et al. 2000), whereas MH is a pharmacogenetic disorder of calcium regulation in skeletal muscle (H. Rosenberg and Fletcher 1994). These contrasting mechanisms also may account for the differential effect of nondepolarizing muscle relaxants, which reduce rigidity in NMS by blocking neural input to muscle receptors but have no effect in MH patients (H. Rosenberg and Fletcher 1994; Sangal and Dimitrijevic 1985).

The similarities in clinical symptoms between NMS and MH have raised practical questions about the risks of cross-reactivity between the syndromes. The available data suggest that patients who develop NMS are not at risk for MH during anesthesia (Caroff et al. 1994a, 1994b, 2001c; Keck et al. 1995). Three reports of fever, rigidity, and rhabdomyolysis occurring after the use of succinylcholine during electroconvulsive treatment of NMS episodes have been published (Grigg 1988; Kelly and Brull 1994; Lazarus and Rosenberg 1991). However, these reactions are not convincing as MH episodes, even though one patient tested positive for MH susceptibility (Lazarus and Rosenberg 1991). Results from other studies of MH susceptibility in groups of NMS patients, in which in vitro skeletal muscle contracture tests were used, have been inconsistent and inconclusive (Adnet et al. 2000; Caroff et al. 1987, 1994a, 1994b).

Epidemiological data provide more convincing evidence that NMS patients are not at risk for MH. NMS patients and their families have been safely anesthetized on repeated occasions with known MH-triggering agents (Geiduschek et al. 1988; Hermesh et al. 1988). In fact, ECT with the use of succinylcholine has been an effective treatment for the acute and residual manifestations of NMS (Caroff et al. 2000c; J.M. Davis et al. 2000).

The converse question—whether patients with MH are at risk for NMS—remains intriguing. MH-susceptible pigs do not appear to be more likely to develop hyperthermia from neuroleptics compared with control animals (Keck et al. 1990; Somers and McLoughlin 1982). In contrast, patients with MH susceptibility have been reported to develop NMS-like reactions after exposure to neuroleptics or other centrally active drugs (Loghmanee and Tobak 1986; Pollock et al. 1992, 1993; Portfl et al. 1999; Sato et al. 1992).

Other evidence suggests that patients with underlying muscle pathology apart from MH have an increased risk of NMS. Calore and colleagues (1994) reported a case of NMS in a patient with central core disease, which is also associated with MH. Schneider et al. (2002) reported a patient with proximal myotonic dystrophy who had a positive in vitro contracture test for MH susceptibility and who experienced muscle stiffness, oculogyric dystonias, and elevated CPK levels following treatment with antipsychotics. An increased risk of NMS has been proposed for patients with elevated baseline levels of CPK or with other evidence of muscle dysfunction (R.J. Downey et al. 1992; Flyckt et al. 2000; Hermesh et al. 1996). In addition,

Miyatake et al. (1996) found a mutation associated with MH susceptibility in the ryanodine receptor in a psychiatric patient with repeated CPK elevations. Finally, neuroleptics have been shown in some studies to have direct effects on CPK levels and membrane permeability, calcium regulation, and contractures in skeletal muscle (Caroff et al. 1994a, 1994b, 2001c; Meltzer et al. 1996). Accordingly, although neuroleptic agents have been considered safe for MH patients (Caroff et al. 1994a; Hon et al. 1991; Lazarus et al. 1989), the above findings suggest some risk of hyperthermic reactions to neuroleptic agents in these patients. With an intrinsic defect in calcium regulation in muscle cells, MH patients may be susceptible to the development of rigidity and hyperthermia when muscle tone and metabolism are stimulated by neuroleptics through either of two mechanisms: 1) neuroleptic-induced increases in neural drive mediated by effects on the extrapyramidal system or 2) direct effects of neuroleptics on skeletal muscle. The same risk may apply to patients with other disorders of muscle function.

Conversely, patients with hypodopaminergia or other central trait vulnerabilities for NMS do not necessarily have skeletal muscle defects associated with susceptibility to MH. Nevertheless, the sensitivity of some patients with MH and other muscle disorders to neuroleptics, the unresolved enigma of CPK elevations in psychiatric patients, and the pharmacological effects of neuroleptics on muscle function are intriguing observations that merit further study in relation to the pathogenesis of NMS.

Animal Models

Several investigators have attempted to develop animal models of NMS. In a series of studies in rats pretreated with haloperidol, Yamawaki and colleagues (Kato and Yamawaki 1989; S. Yamawaki et al. 1990a) sought to simulate an NMS-like disorder by the stereotactic microinjection of veratrine, a sodium-channel modulator, into the preoptic anterior hypothalamus. This resulted in hyperthermia, abnormal behaviors, and increased turnover of dopamine and serotonin. Because this effect could be inhibited by serotonin antagonists, S. Yamawaki et al. (1990a) and Kato and Yamawaki (1989) concluded that hyperthermia in NMS reflected a relative increase in serotoninergic activity over dopamine thermoregulatory centers. However, this may be difficult to reconcile with reports of reduced serotonin metabolites in the CSF during NMS (Nisijima and Ishiguro 1990, 1995a).

Parada et al. (1995) injected sulpiride in the periformical lateral hypothalamus in rats, resulting in increased intracranial temperature, which could be attenuated by dopamine. Apart from intracranial temperature elevations, this appears to bear an incomplete resemblance to NMS. A more complete model was proposed by Tanii et al. (1996), who administered haloperidol and atropine to rabbits during exposure to high ambient temperature (35°C). They observed significant increases in muscle rigidity and electromyographic activity, serum CPK levels, and body temperature, which were normalized by administration of dantrolene.

Several investigators have studied animal models of MH to ascertain the mechanisms underlying NMS. Somers and McLoughlin (1982) observed that neuroleptics actually delayed the onset of rigidity in halothane-sensitive MH pigs. Keck et al. (1990) conducted unique studies in MH-susceptible pigs to test whether this could be a viable model for NMS. They found that lithium and haloperidol administered together, but not separately, induced the porcine stress syndrome in two of three susceptible and one of three nonsusceptible pigs. They concluded that the MH model in pigs was not entirely consistent with NMS, although lithium has been proposed as an additional risk factor for NMS in humans (Caroff and Mann 1993; Lazarus et al. 1989).

However, the animal models for MH may offer an opportunity to study stress-sensitive mechanisms in relation to neurotransmitters involved in NMS. Draper et al. (1984) reported that stress-susceptible pigs had a 20%–40% baseline reduction of dopamine in the caudate nucleus compared with normal pigs, suggesting that MH may reflect hypodopaminergic mechanisms in these animals. As reviewed by Wappler et al. (2001), in vivo studies in stress-susceptible pigs have found that administration of 5-HT_2 receptor agonists can initiate the MH syndrome, which can be blocked by pretreatment with serotonin antagonists. These latter findings also may be difficult to reconcile with reduced levels of central serotonin metabolites observed in cases of NMS and may serve as a better model for cases of serotonin syndrome.

🗝 Conclusion

NMS is an uncommon but potentially fatal reaction associated with the use of dopamine antagonists in the treatment of psychoses and other disorders. Although increased awareness has resulted in probable declines in incidence and mortality, clinical vigilance remains important in diagnosis and treatment.

NMS occurs in approximately 0.2% of patients who start or restart taking antipsychotics. Proposed risk factors include previous NMS episodes, dehydration, agitation, dose of medication, and the rate and route of administration. Although NMS has been reported in association with new atypical antipsychotics, the incidence of the disorder with these agents may be reduced. Although NMS has been reported in patients with diverse psychiatric diagnoses as well as in persons without psychiatric illnesses, patients with organic brain disorders, schizophrenia, mood disorders, or catatonia may be at increased risk. These risk factors for NMS do not outweigh the potential benefits of antipsychotic therapy in most patients.

Early recognition and diagnosis are key to a successful outcome. In most cases, the onset of NMS is characterized by changes in mental status or the development of catatonia or extrapyramidal rigidity. Hypermetabolism and hyperthermia generally develop later in the course of the syndrome. Standardized criteria for the diagnosis of NMS have been developed and emphasize the classic findings of hyperthermia, muscle rigidity, mental status changes, and autonomic dysfunction. In uncomplicated cases, the syndrome lasts 7–10 days in those receiving oral neuroleptics. The duration of illness can be prolonged in association with depot drugs or in cases in which residual catatonic and parkinsonian signs persist.

Treatment consists primarily of early recognition, discontinuation of triggering drugs, management of fluid balance, temperature reduction, and monitoring for complications. Substantial theoretical and clinical experience supports trials of benzodiazepines, dopamine agonists, dantrolene, or ECT. These specific treatments should be considered empirically and chosen based on the character, severity, and duration of NMS symptoms in an individual patient. As a result of these measures, mortality from NMS has declined in recent years, although fatalities still occur. Neuroleptics may be safely reintroduced in the management of most patients who have recovered from an NMS episode, although a significant risk of recurrence does exist, dependent in part on time elapsed since recovery and dose or potency of neuroleptics used.

The differential diagnosis of NMS is complex and challenging. Although it encompasses a broad range of febrile disorders, NMS is most difficult to distinguish from, and most fascinating to compare with, other hypermetabolic and stress-related disorders encountered in clinical practice. Although these disorders appear to differ in triggering mechanisms, they culminate in a final common pathway of systemic hypermetabolic activity and hyperthermia.

Direct evidence from physiological and neuroanatomical measures and indirect evidence obtained from pharmacological experience and comparisons with Parkinson's disease clearly indicate the importance of trait and state-related reductions in central dopamine activity in the pathogenesis of NMS. However, additional studies of NMS in patients, animal models, and pharmacological mechanisms may lead to innovative risk reduction strategies and the optimization and increasing safety of antipsychotic therapy.

CHAPTER 2

Thermoregulatory Mechanisms and Antipsychotic Drug–Related Heatstroke

Along with neuroleptic malignant syndrome (NMS), two additional hyperthermic syndromes have been described in association with antipsychotic drug treatment: so-called benign hyperthermia and antipsychotic drug–related heatstroke (ADRHS). Benign hyperthermia has been viewed as a hypersensitivity reaction or, alternatively, as the product of mild antipsychotic drug–induced thermoregulatory impairment (Belfer and Shader 1970). It develops during the first 3 weeks of treatment, is usually associated with mild temperature elevation, and is brief. Benign hyperthermia has been reported in 0.7%–5.7% of patients beginning antipsychotic drug treatment (Kick 1981) but occurs in 10%–20% (Meltzer 1992) or more (Nitenson et al. 1995) of those starting clozapine. Clozapine has been shown to stimulate the release of pyrogenic cytokines (Pollmacher et al. 1997), including tumor necrosis factor α (TNF-α), a cytokine that is likely to play an important role in clozapine-induced benign hyperthermia and in that drug's hematopoietic side effects, including agranulocytosis (Pollmacher et al. 2000). Temperature elevations well above 38.5°C have been observed in some clozapine-treated patients. When this occurs, clozapine should be discontinued and other causes of hyperthermia, including NMS and infections secondary to agranulocytosis, ruled out (van Kammen and Marder 1995).

In contrast to benign hyperthermia, ADRHS and NMS represent potentially lethal complications of antipsychotic drug treatment. Both disorders appear underrecognized, share some clinical features, and may be confused with a host of other hyperthermic illnesses, including serotonin syndrome (Chapter 3) and fulminating hyperthermic syndromes related to therapy with or abuse of a wide array of other psychotropic agents (see Chapter 4). Furthermore, both ADRHS and NMS resemble clinical descriptions of non-drug-related malignant catatonia (Chapter 5).

In this chapter, we review the physiology of normal thermoregulation and present data indicating a key role for dopamine in central thermoregulatory heat-loss mechanisms. Despite diverse pharmacological activities, all antipsychotics, both typical agents (neuroleptics) and the newer atypical drugs, block a relevant number of dopamine receptors. Accordingly, these data suggest that antipsychotics can promote hyperthermia by interrupting dopamine-mediated heat-loss pathways in a hot environment or during excessive endogenous heat production. Furthermore, substantial evidence also supports the involvement of serotonin in central thermoregulation and points to its participation in dopamine-mediated heat loss. On the other hand, serotonin has been implicated in hyperthermic responses, as in serotonin syndrome. The potential for differential thermoregulatory effects of atypical antipsychotics compared with typical agents is considered in light of the spectrum of serotoninergic receptors with which these newer drugs interact.

We emphasize the concept of "fever" as a discrete subtype of hyperthermia differing physiologically from other types of body temperature elevation resulting from pathological or pharmacological impairment of thermoregulatory mechanisms. We describe the clinical presentation of heatstroke and review the social, behavioral, and medical factors that place psychiatric patients at risk for heatstroke. We also explore not only the role of antipsychotic drug effects on central dopaminergic and serotoninergic pathways in the etiology of ADRHS but also the contribution of peripheral anticholinergic activity of antipsychotics themselves or of anticholinergic drugs administered concurrently.

🔊 Normal Thermoregulation

Warm-blooded animals are generally able to maintain body temperature within narrow limits despite large variations in ambient temperature (Bruck 1989; Guyton and Hall 2000; Schafer 1998). This is accomplished by a highly effective homeostatic control system in which peripheral and core thermosensors monitor the body's thermal state and transmit information to a hypothalamic central controller (Figure 2–1). Here, converging central and peripheral temperature signals are integrated and compared with the "set point." The set point represents an optimal steady-state temperature at which no thermoregulatory responses are activated. If the controller detects a change in body temperature away from the set point, it activates autonomic and behavioral thermoregulatory effectors to counteract that change. The set point is generally conceptualized as an endogenous reference signal generated independent of core body temperature by neurons located within the central nervous system (CNS) interface between thermosensors and thermoeffectors.

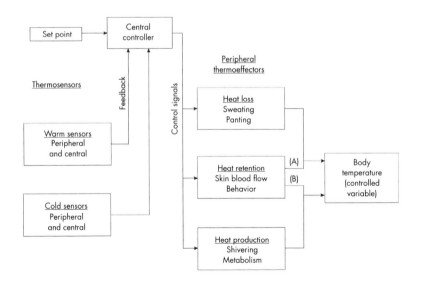

(A) Contributes to reduction of bodily heat when either central or peripheral temperature rises above the thermoneutral zone.

(B) Contributes to increase of bodily heat when either central or peripheral temperature falls below the thermoneutral zone.

FIGURE 2–1.   Block diagram of thermoregulation.

Source.   Adapted from Bruck K: "Thermal Balance and the Regulation of Body Temperature," in *Human Physiology.* Edited by Schmidt RF, Thews G. Berlin, Germany, Springer-Verlag, 1989, pp. 624–644. Used with permission.

The preoptic and anterior hypothalamus (PO/AH) and nearby circumventricular and septal regions represent the most important components in the central thermoregulatory system and are the first structures to detect and respond to a departure of body temperature away from the set point (Boulant 1996; Satinoff 1978). Electrophysiological studies show that some PO/AH neurons are thermosensitive, not only sensing hypothalamic temperature but also receiving afferent input from thermoreceptors in skin and spinal cord (Boulant 1994, 1996). These neurons, therefore, are capable of integrating central and peripheral thermal information, and this integration allows the selection of thermoregulatory responses that are appropriate for the internal and external thermal conditions. Although other CNS thermoregulatory sites throughout the brain and spinal cord are capable of integrating local and peripheral thermal information, the PO/AH serves to coordinate and adjust the activity of these lower centers. Without its input, thermoregulatory responses at the most caudal sites would be activated only at extremely hot or cold temperatures.

Studies have identified three major types of PO/AH neurons: warm-sensitive neurons, cold-sensitive neurons, and temperature-insensitive neurons. Increases in hypothalamic temperature produce increased firing rates in warm-sensitive neurons and decreased firing rates in cold-sensitive neurons. Both in vivo and in vitro studies find that about 30% of PO/AH neurons are warm sensitive, fewer than 10% are cold sensitive, and more than 60% are temperature insensitive (Boulant et al. 1997). Temperature-insensitive neurons act as constant reference input to effector neurons, and this provides the basis for the set point temperature. Warm-sensitive neurons may be divided into three groups based on their ranges of firing rates at 38°C: low-firing, medium-firing, and high-firing neurons (Boulant 1996). Boulant (1994, 1996) suggested that cold-sensitive neurons are not inherently thermosensitive but, rather, derive their preoptic neuronal cold sensitivity from synaptic inhibition by nearby warm-sensitive hypothalamic neurons.

Figure 2–2 provides a neuronal model of how PO/AH neurons may integrate central and peripheral thermal signals, activating effector mechanisms for heat loss and heat gain. The lowest-firing warm-sensitive neurons express their hypothalamic thermosensitivity in the hyperthermic range. Accordingly, their most likely thermoregulatory role would be to control heat-loss responses such as panting and, particularly in humans, sweating that are operative only when the PO/AH is warmed above the thermoneutral range (Boulant 1996). As indicated in Figure 2–2, it appears that these neurons have low firing rates because they receive a minimal amount of excitatory input from peripheral warm receptors.

Medium-firing warm-sensitive neurons are equally thermosensitive above and below the normal PO/AH temperature, and their most likely

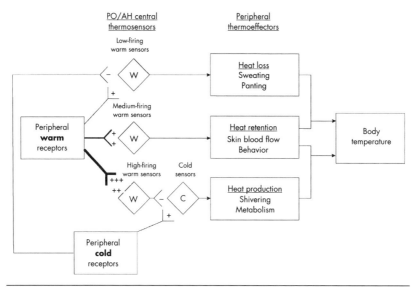

FIGURE 2–2. Neuronal model of thermoregulation.

Note. PO/AH=preoptic and anterior hypothalamus.
Source. Adapted from Boulant JA: "Hypothalamic Neurons Regulating Body Temperature," in *Handbook of Physiology, Section 4: Environmental Physiology: A Critical, Comprehensive Presentation of Physiological Knowledge and Concepts,* Two Volume Set. Edited by Fregly MJ, Blatteis CM. New York, Oxford University Press, 1996, pp. 105–126. Copyright 1996 American Physiological Society. Used by permission of Oxford University Press, Inc.

thermoregulatory role would be to control heat-retention responses such as skin blood flow and thermoregulatory behavior. Heat-retention responses are most active in the thermoneutral range and represent the first effector mechanisms recruited when body temperature is altered above or below the set point (Boulant 1996). Medium-firing warm-sensitive neurons receive a moderate amount of excitatory input from peripheral warm receptors, and this probably accounts for their medium firing rates. Skin blood flow is the principal autonomic thermoeffector mechanism involved in heat retention. In addition, heat retention is maintained by thermoregulatory behavior, such as fanning oneself or adding or removing clothing. The PO/AH has both afferent and efferent connections with various limbic areas and pathways that participate in emotional coloring of sensory input. These limbic components evaluate afferent information from thermoreceptors as "thermally" comfortable or uncomfortable and initiate compensatory behavioral responses. As such, it is of considerable interest that, in vivo, much of the excitatory input to medium-firing warm-sensitive neurons comes from the hippocampus, a limbic structure linked with emotion, behavior, and memory (Boulant 1996).

Because their spontaneous firing rate is near its maximal sustainable level, high-firing warm-sensitive receptors do not show a further increase in firing rate during PO/AH warming. Rather, they express their greatest thermosensitivity during PO/AH cooling, at which time they decrease their rate of firing. The most likely thermoregulatory role of high-firing warm-sensitive receptors would be to control heat-production responses that occur in the hypothermic range: nonshivering thermogenesis and, in humans, primarily shivering thermogenesis. As illustrated in Figure 2–2, high-firing warm-sensitive neurons receive a great amount of excitatory input from peripheral warm receptors. This figure also indicates that nearby, tonically active cold-sensitive neurons receive synaptic inhibition from high-firing warm-sensitive neurons. Accordingly, PO/AH cooling decreases inhibition from high-firing warm-sensitive neurons, thus increasing the firing rate of cold-sensitive neurons and further activating heat-production responses. In addition, PO/AH cold-sensitive neurons are affected by peripheral cold receptors (Boulant 1996).

In humans, sweating and increased skin blood flow, along with behavioral modifications, are the thermoeffector mechanisms active at high ambient temperatures. Three major avenues are available for dissipation of bodily heat: 1) radiation of heat through space, 2) convection and conduction to air currents, and 3) evaporation of sweat (Guyton and Hall 2000). Heat loss to air currents reaches a maximum as wind velocity approaches 15–20 miles per hour, and evaporation is facilitated by a dry environment. As the ambient temperature approaches that of the body, radiation, convection, and conduction will yield a net heat gain rather than a heat loss, leaving evaporation as the only mechanism of heat loss. Sweat glands, under the control of sympathetic nerves that have muscarinic endings rather than adrenergic endings, provide water to be vaporized by the heat brought to the body surface by dilated peripheral vessels. However, high humidity will impair this mechanism because less sweat can be lost to the already highly saturated air. Thus, continuous heat storage may occur in a hot, windless, and humid environment. Because vulnerability to heat storage may be offset by acclimatization, which requires several weeks of exposure to heat to develop, sudden rises in ambient temperature during heat waves can present a particular problem.

🗐 Dopamine and Serotonin in Thermoregulation

In 1971, Bligh et al. proposed a model for the involvement of monoamines in mammalian hypothalamic thermoregulation (Figure 2–3). Data were derived through intracerebroventricular (ICV) injection of serotonin, acetylcholine, and norepinephrine in sheep, goats, and rabbits. Two principal pathways between thermoreceptors and thermoregulators were described. One was from warm sensors to heat-loss effectors and the other from cold sensors to heat-production effectors. Because heat production is reduced by exposure to heat, and heat loss is reduced by exposure to cold, crossed inhibitory pathways were included between the two main pathways. In this model, serotonin acts along the pathway from warm sensors to heat-loss effectors, activating heat-loss mechanisms of panting and vasodilatation and inhibiting shivering. Acetylcholine acts along the pathway from cold sensors to heat-production effectors, activating shivering, causing vasoconstriction, and decreasing panting. Norepinephrine functions as an inhibitor between the two main pathways, suppressing all thermoeffector mechanisms active at a given ambient temperature.

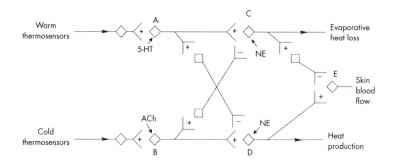

FIGURE 2–3. Role of serotonin (5-HT), norepinephrine (NE), and acetylcholine (Ach) in the control of body temperature in sheep.

Source. Adapted from Bligh J, Cottle WH, Maskrey M: "Influence of Ambient Temperature on the Thermoregulatory Responses to 5-Hydroxytryptamine, Noradrenaline and Acetylcholine Injections Into the Lateral Cerebral Ventricles of Sheep, Goats and Rabbits." *Journal of Physiology* 212:377–392, 1971. Used with permission.

Dopamine was not included in the Bligh et al. (1971) model. Pharmacological support for a role for dopamine in central thermoregulation originated from evidence that central and systemic injections of specific dopamine agonists such as apomorphine and amantadine could lower body temperature in rodents, a response that could be blocked by specific dopamine antagonists such as pimozide (Cox and Lee 1977; Cox and Tha 1975). Dopamine agonist–induced hypothermia was found to be ambient temperature dependent; dose-related decreases in body temperature occurred at 20°C or below, whereas hyperthermia developed at 29°C (Lin 1979). Similar work in sheep and goats indicated that ICV injection of dopamine caused hypothermia, which was also blocked by dopamine antagonists (De Roij et al. 1977, 1978a). Moreover, amphetamine, an indirect dopamine agonist, caused a similar hypothermia in rats maintained at low ambient temperatures (Yehuda and Wurtman 1975). In these studies, however, agents were administered either systemically or intracerebroventricularly, leaving their exact site of action unclear. Also, experiments involving dopamine agonists and antagonists relied heavily on the assumption that these agents were not simply acting on noradrenergic receptors (Cox and Lee 1980). Furthermore, these investigations failed to demonstrate the physiological involvement of endogenous dopamine in the central thermoregulatory mediation of heat loss because in order to elicit hypothermia, they had been performed at or below room temperature, where such an endogenous heat-loss system probably would be quiescent.

Following reports involving intrahypothalamic injections of dopamine in the rat (Cox and Lee 1980; Cox et al. 1978) and cat (Ruwe and Myers 1978), a precise anatomical delineation of dopamine-sensitive sites emerged (T.F. Lee et al. 1985). The most sensitive site for dopamine-mediated hypothermia was localized to a specific region of the PO/AH, the key hypothalamic thermoregulatory area. Furthermore, Cox and Lee (1980) and Ruwe and Myers (1978) were able to identify in the rat and cat, respectively, PO/AH norepinephrine-sensitive sites located away from the dopamine-sensitive sites, confirming that dopamine agonists do not cause hypothermia through actions on noradrenergic mechanisms.

In further studies, Cox and associates (Cox and Lee 1980; Cox et al. 1978) were able to confirm a physiological role for endogenous dopamine as a central mediator of heat loss by using bilateral injections of the dopamine antagonists pimozide and haloperidol into the PO/AH of rats exposed to an infrared lamp–imposed heat load. Under such circumstances, an endogenous heat-loss system would be expected to be activated. Prior to dopamine antagonist treatment, rats responded to the imposed heat load by vasodilatation of tail skin blood vessels, yielding an increase in tail skin temperature but little increase in core body temperature. Following dopamine antagonist treatment, rats had a reduced rise in tail temperature on heat exposure and a significant elevation in core body temperature, consistent with physiological involvement of endogenous dopamine in the mediation of heat loss. Further studies by this group of investigators indicated that dopamine plays a far more prominent role than norepinephrine in PO/AH heat-loss mechanisms. Furthermore, electrophysiological studies examining the firing rate and thermosensitivity of individual PO/AH neurons perfused with dopamine have shown that dopamine excites a large portion of warm-sensitive neurons and inhibits cold-sensitive neurons (Scott and Boulant 1984).

In the Bligh et al. (1971) model, serotonin mediates heat loss and acts along the pathway from warm sensors to heat-loss effectors. De Roij et al. (1978b) provided evidence for the involvement of serotonin in dopamine-mediated hypothermia. They noted that in goats maintained at an ambient temperature of 20°C, ICV injections of both dopamine and serotonin caused a decreased core body temperature and dilatation of ear vessels. Whereas the thermoregulatory response at 20°C to ICV administration of dopamine could be blocked by both the dopamine antagonist haloperidol and the serotonin antagonist methysergide, the thermoregulatory response to ICV serotonin could be blocked by only methysergide. These findings suggested that dopamine-mediated hypothermia is the product of primary dopaminergic stimulation, resulting in a secondary release of serotonin, which activates the heat-loss mechanisms. Cox et al. (1980) were able to localize such a dopamine/serotonin link in the rat to the previously identified dopamine-sensitive site for hypothermia within the PO/AH. Similar to findings in the goat, a report by Cox et al. (1980) found that methysergide in the rat reduced the hypothermic response to central injection of both dopamine and serotonin, whereas haloperidol blocked only the response to dopamine.

The accumulated evidence suggested that dopamine should replace norepinephrine in at least some of the hypothalamic synapses occupied by norepinephrine in the original Bligh et al. (1971) model of mammalian thermoregulation. Consistent with the previous discussion, a likely location at which dopamine could act as an excitatory neurotransmitter mediating heat loss would be in the pathway from warm sensors to heat-loss effectors before the serotonin synapse (Cox et al. 1978, 1980; De Roij et al. 1978b). This proposed revision of the Bligh et al. (1971) model is shown in Figure 2–4. Although the cell bodies of the serotonin-containing neurons are probably located in the midbrain raphe nuclei, it seems likely that dopamine acts on their nerve terminals in the PO/AH.

Along with the PO/AH, the nigrostriatal dopamine system may be involved in dopamine-mediated heat-loss mechanisms (T. F. Lee et al. 1985). Bilateral apomorphine injections into the substantia nigra of the rat produced a dose-related hypothermia that was almost identical in magnitude and time course to the same dose of apomorphine injected bilaterally into the PO/AH (S. J. Brown et al. 1982). Hypothermia was blocked by bilateral injections of pimozide into the substantia nigra. Furthermore, bilateral electrolytic lesioning of the substantia nigra has been associated with significant hyperthermia in rats exposed to heat (S. J. Brown et al. 1982). Thus, the substantia nigra might represent a "lower" thermoregulatory center (Satinoff 1978) caudal to the PO/AH, as discussed earlier. Consistent with this schema, the substantia nigra would be expected to transmit thermoregulatory impulses to the more rostral PO/AH, in addition to its

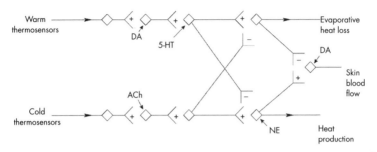

FIGURE 2–4. Incorporation of dopamine (DA) in the neuronal model of thermoregulation.

Note. 5-HT=serotonin; Ach=acetylcholine; NE=norepinephrine.
Source. Reprinted from De Roij TAJM, Frens J, Woutersen-Van Nijanten F, et al.: "Comparison of Thermoregulatory Responses to Intracerebroventricularly Injected Dopamine, Noradrenaline and 5-Hydroxytryptamine in the Goat." *European Journal of Pharmacology* 49: 395–405, 1978b. Used with permission. Copyright 1978 Elsevier Science.

local role in thermoregulation. Alternatively, the major thermoregulatory role of the substantia nigra may involve activation of heat-loss mechanisms in response to impulses from the PO/AH (T.F. Lee et al. 1985) transmitted through a pathway from the PO/AH to the substantia nigra, as described by Swanson (1976). T.F. Lee and associates (1985) have suggested that transmission from the substantia nigra to the midbrain reticular formation could influence autonomic mechanisms for heat loss, whereas nigrostriatal projections to the thalamus, and ultimately to motor cortex, could facilitate behavioral heat loss.

It was originally suggested that hypothermic responses to dopamine agonists in the rat, as well as several other animal species, were mediated exclusively through D_2 dopamine receptors (Faunt and Crocker 1987; Hjorth and Carlsson 1988). Studies that used the D_1 dopamine receptor agonist SKF 38393 indicated that this receptor was not involved. However, conclusions were limited in that SKF 38393 appears to be a partial agonist at the D_1 dopamine receptor and that the relatively high dosages used in temperature studies could not exclude nonspecific effects of the drug. Later work indicated that although hypothermia appears mediated primarily by D_2 dopamine receptors, D_1 receptors might exert a modulatory role (Nunes et al. 1991; Verma and Kulkarni 1993). More recently, Salmi and associates (Salmi 1998; Salmi et al. 1993) provided evidence that both D_1 and D_2 receptors are specifically involved in causing hypothermia in the rat. Salmi et al. (1993) used the selective full D_1 dopamine agonist A 68930 to produce a hypothermic response in the rat that was antagonized by the selective D_1 antagonist SCH 23390 but not by the selective D_2 antagonist raclopride. In contrast, hypothermia induced by the D_2 agonist quinpirole was antagonized by raclopride but not SCH 23390 treatment. Hypothermia produced by both receptor subtypes appears mediated by postsynaptic dopamine receptors (Ahlenius and Salmi 1994). In further support of the involvement of D_1 receptors in hypothermia, dihydrexidine, another selective full D_1 receptor agonist, also resulted in SCH 23390–sensitive hypothermia in rats (Salmi 1998; Salmi and Ahlenius 1997). Taken together, these observations provide strong evidence for a specific and independent role of D_1 dopamine receptors in heat-loss mechanisms in rats, distinct from effects mediated via D_2 dopamine receptors.

In addition to D_1 and D_2 receptors, novel D_3, D_4, and D_5 dopamine receptor subtypes have been cloned. D_3 dopamine receptors (Sokoloff et al. 1990) also may participate in hypothermic mechanisms. In general, both typical and atypical antipsychotics manifest a slight to modest preference for D_2 over D_3 receptors (Schwartz et al. 2000). Millan et al. (1994, 1995) studied a series of dopamine agonists with affinity for both D_3 and D_2 receptors and found that their ability to evoke hypothermia corresponded to their relative affinity at D_3 rather than D_2 receptors. Furthermore, as compared with mildly preferential D_3 dopamine antagonists, the highly preferential D_3 antagonist S 14297 potently and selectively abolished the hypothermia elicited by the D_3 preferential agonist 7-OH-DPAT. Finally, across all antagonists, potency for inhibition of the induction of hypothermia by 7-OH-DPAT correlated more powerfully with affinities at D_3 than D_2 receptors. Although not fully excluding a role for D_2 receptors, these data suggest that D_3 dopamine receptors are of primary importance in mediating hypothermia in the rat (Millan et al. 1994, 1995). The investigators further concluded that a role for D_4 or D_5 in the mediation of hypothermia is unlikely.

Recently, Perachon et al. (2000) questioned evidence derived from the finding of S 14297 reversal of 7-OH-DPAT–induced hypothermia, when both compounds are considered preferential D_3 receptor ligands, and they challenged the notion that D_3 dopamine receptors play a primary role in dopamine agonist–induced hypothermia. These investigators found that 7-OH-DPAT does not act as a selective D_3 agonist in functional tests in vitro. Furthermore, based on in vitro functional studies, they showed that S 14297 functions as a full D_3 agonist rather than a D_3 antagonist. In addition, they showed that S 14297 is a partial agonist at the D_2 receptor. This suggested that antagonism of 7-OH-DPAT–induced hypothermia by S 14297 might be the result of its D_2 partial agonist activity rather than the previously proposed agonism at D_3 receptors. Furthermore, regarding Millan and associates' (1994, 1995) observation that the potencies of a series of dopamine agonists in inducing hypothermia correlate better with their affinity for D_3

than D_2 receptors, Perachon et al. (2000) underscored that in vitro activity is a poor indicator of the functional potency of agonists at D_2 and D_3 receptors. In functional studies in which the most preferential D_3 agonists available were used, they found significant correlations between hypothermia and both D_2 and D_3 receptors. Furthermore, this hypothermia was reversed by antagonists with a rank order of potency more typical of the D_2 than the D_3 receptor. Finally, the absence of significant changes in the potency and efficacy of 7-OH-DPAT to elicit hypothermia in mice lacking D_3 receptors also supports the view that this receptor is not necessary for dopamine agonist–induced hypothermia. The latter is consistent with the failure of Boulay et al. (1999) to find differences in dopamine receptor agonist–induced hypothermia between D_3 receptor knockout mice and control mice. Taken together, these findings suggest that hypothermia does not result from a selective stimulation of D_3 receptors and indicate that D_1, D_2, and D_3 receptors all play prominent roles in dopamine-mediated heat-loss mechanisms.

Although, as considered previously, a role for serotonin in dopamine receptor–mediated thermoregulatory mechanisms has been suggested, similar uncertainty exists regarding the involvement of distinct serotonin receptors in thermoregulatory heat-loss pathways. Administration of serotonin agonists has been shown to produce differential, as well as marked, changes in the body temperature of the rat depending on the agent and route of administration (Gudelsky et al. 1986; Lin et al. 1998). Behavioral studies in rodents have focused on the functional consequences of activating various subtypes of serotonin receptors. For example, the head-twitch response in mice and its behavioral homologue, the "wet-dog" shakes in rats, appear mediated by serotonin type 2A ($5\text{-}HT_{2A}$) receptors. On the other hand, behavioral studies across several animal species suggest that many features of the serotonin syndrome appear related to overstimulation of the postsynaptic $5\text{-}HT_{1A}$ receptors, although hyperthermia seems mediated by different serotonin receptor subtypes. In fact, the $5\text{-}HT_{1A}$ receptor agonist 8-OH-DPAT induces hypothermia in rodents, and this hypothermic effect can be blocked by the $5\text{-}HT_{1A}$ antagonist WAY 100635. Of note, there are species differences in the mechanisms underlying the hypothermic effect of $5\text{-}HT_{1A}$ receptor agonists: in the mouse, it appears presynaptic, whereas in the rat, it can be mediated both pre- and postsynaptically (Barnes and Sharp 1999). As such, it now appears increasingly likely that the serotonin receptor that mediates hypothermia and is linked to dopamine in the Bligh et al. (1971) model's pathway from warm sensors to heat-loss effectors is of the $5\text{-}HT_{1A}$ subtype.

In contrast, hyperthermia is produced in both rodents and humans by serotonin agonists, such as (+/–)-1-(2,5-dimethoxy-4-iodophenyl)-2-aminopropane HCL (DOI), quipazine, and MK-212, that directly activate

5-HT$_{2A/2C}$ receptors (Lin et al. 1998; Salmi and Ahlenius 1998; S. Yamawaki et al. 1983). Furthermore, hyperthermia induced by these agents can be antagonized by pretreatment with the 5-HT$_{2A/2C}$ receptor antagonists ritanserin and ketanserin. Studies of the selective 5-HT$_{2A}$ antagonist amperozide suggest that 5-HT$_{2A}$ receptors may be key in mediating hyperthermia in the rat, and activation of these receptors appears implicated in the hyperthermia of serotonin syndrome (Nisijima et al. 2001). Of note, some studies have reported hypothermia during treatment with 5-HT$_{2A}$ antagonists alone (Cryan et al. 2000; Gudelsky et al. 1986), although others have not (Salmi and Ahlenius 1998). Furthermore, data from studies of D-fenfluramine-induced thermoregulatory changes in the rat suggest that 5-HT$_{2C}$ receptor stimulation may result in hypothermia (Cryan et al. 2000). These data support further additions to the Bligh et al. (1971) model, with a 5-HT$_{2A}$ receptor now included in the hyperthermia pathway from cold sensors to heat-production effectors, and the postulation of a 5-HT$_{2C}$ receptor in the upper heat-loss pathway.

Our review of the potential involvement of distinct dopamine and serotonin receptor subtypes in heat-loss and heat-production pathways supports further revisions in the Bligh et al. (1971) model of mammalian thermoregulation. The implications of the present data are presented in Figure 2–5. In addition to D$_2$ dopamine receptors, D$_1$ and D$_3$ dopamine receptors appear likely to participate in the heat-loss pathway from warm receptors to heat-production effectors. Furthermore, the proposed dopamine/serotonin hypothermic link is now indicated as mediated by 5-HT$_{1A}$ receptors, primarily of the postsynaptic type. In addition, a tentative role for 5-HT$_{2C}$ receptors in mediating heat loss is suggested. As discussed previously, this upper heat-loss pathway would be physiologically active only at high environmental temperatures. Excitatory 5-HT$_{2A}$ receptors are now posited to be located in the heat-production pathway, from cold sensors to heat-production effectors. Conversely, this pathway would be physiologically active only at low environmental temperatures. Although highly speculative, our revisions to the Bligh et al. (1971) model are supported by the recent work of Cryan et al. (2000), characterizing the serotonin and dopamine receptor subtypes mediating the hypo- and hyperthermic effects of fenfluramine.

🌀 Atypical Antipsychotic Drugs and Specific Dopamine and Serotonin Receptor Subtypes: Implications for Thermoregulatory Effects

Such an expanded view of the participation of diverse dopamine and serotonin receptors in the Bligh model provides insight into the numerous ways

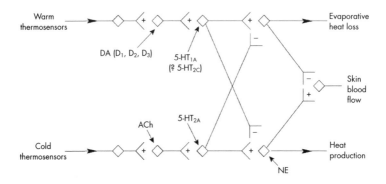

FIGURE 2–5. Incorporation of distinct dopamine (DA) and serotonin (5-HT) receptor subtypes in the neuronal model of thermoregulation.

Note. Ach=acetylcholine; NE=norepinephrine.

Source. Adapted from Bligh J, Cottle WH, Maskrey M: "Influence of Ambient Temperature on the Thermoregulatory Responses to 5-Hydroxytryptamine, Noradrenaline and Acetylcholine Injections Into the Lateral Cerebral Ventricles of Sheep, Goats and Rabbits." *Journal of Physiology* 212:377–392, 1971. Used with permission.

that the new group of atypical or novel antipsychotics may affect thermoregulation. A uniform observation in studies of mammalian thermoregulation has been that antipsychotic drugs promote poikilothermia; that is, they render animals thermally dependent on their environment, leading to hypothermia in the cold and hyperthermia in the heat (Kollias and Bullard 1964). Departures from this pattern cluster around studies defining hot and cold ambient temperatures close to thermoneutrality. Given the consistent finding of antipsychotic drug-induced hyperthermia in the heat, and the prominent role of endogenous dopamine in hypothalamic mediation of heat loss, we had proposed that typical or conventional antipsychotics promote hyperthermia by blocking D_2 dopamine receptors (Lazarus et al. 1989; Mann et al. 1991).

The receptor profiles of atypical antipsychotics differ from those of typical agents in several ways. Although considerable variation exists, currently available atypical antipsychotics share the property of reduced affinity for the D_2 dopamine receptor. Risperidone and olanzapine achieve robust antipsychotic activity only at doses that occupy 65% or more of D_2 receptors, the range obtained by low-dose typical antipsychotics (Kapur et al. 1999; Seeman and Tallerico 1999). Although therapeutic dosages of clozapine and quetiapine may occupy up to 70% of D_2 receptors between 2 and 4 hours after a dose, occupancies of only 0%–50% are observed at 12 hours (Seeman 2001; Seeman and Tallerico 1999). This appears due to the fast dissociation of these latter two agents from the D_2 dopamine receptor (Kapur and Seeman 2001). Still, all antipsychotics, typical or atypical, block a relevant number of D_2 receptors and, through this mechanism, could impair heat loss with resultant hyperthermia. In support of this, the atypical antipsychotics olanzapine, quetiapine, and risperidone all have been shown to antagonize hypothermia induced by the selective D_2 dopamine agonist quinpirole in the rat (Oerther and Ahlenius 2000). As discussed later in this section, the failure of clozapine to attenuate hypothermia was attributed to that agent's own strong propensity to lower body temperature at the dosage and ambient temperature used in this study (Heh et al. 1988; Oerther and Ahlenius 2000).

In general, most antipsychotics currently in use bind to both D_1 and D_2 dopamine receptors; no clear correlation has been established between the atypical nature of an antipsychotic and its D_1 affinity. Similarly, both typical and atypical antipsychotic drugs have considerable affinity for D_3 receptors in vitro, with most agents showing a slight to modest preference for the D_2 over the D_3 receptors. Thus, although antipsychotic drug–induced blockade of both D_1 and D_3 receptors appears involved in the propensity of these agents to impair heat loss in a hot environment (in an additive fashion with D_2 receptor blockade) (Figure 2–5), the profile of atypical agents in inducing hyperthermia would appear similar to that of typical antipsychotics in this regard. The role of D_4 and D_5 receptors in antipsychotic drug–induced impairment of heat loss may be limited (Millan et al. 1994, 1995).

Of considerable interest, a recent series of experiments provided evidence that clozapine has D_1 dopamine receptor agonist properties and can produce *hypothermia* in the rat (Oerther and Ahlenius 2000; Salmi and Ahlenius 1996; Salmi et al. 1994). At an ambient temperature of $23.7 \pm 1.5°C$, clozapine produced a robust decrease in body temperature in the rat that was fully antagonized by the selective D_1 receptor antagonist SCH 23390. The atypical agents olanzapine, risperidone, and quetiapine also induced hypothermia at this ambient temperature, but this was not antagonized by SCH 23390. In contrast, hypothermia produced by the D_2 selective agonist quinpirole was at least partially antagonized by olanzapine, risperidone, and quetiapine but not by clozapine. Thus, these authors reported that clozapine showed D_1 dopamine receptor partial agonist properties at low doses at which no D_2 dopamine receptor antagonism was detectable. Conversely, there was no evidence for D_1 dopamine receptor partial agonism with olanzapine, risperidone, or quetiapine at dosages adequate to produce hypothermia (Oerther and Ahlenius 2000).

The same experimental model (i.e., rat core temperature) also found that the D_2 dopamine receptor antagonist raclopride produced a partial antagonism of clozapine-induced hypothermia (Salmi and Ahlenius 1996). This suggests that clozapine also has weak agonist properties at the D_2 dopamine receptor. Other researchers have provided evidence that clozapine is a partial agonist at both D_1 and D_2 dopamine receptors (Jackson et al. 1998; Ninan and Kulkarni 1998). Furthermore, other work suggests that although olanzapine does not show agonism at the D_1 dopamine receptor, it behaves as a D_2 dopamine partial agonist (Ninan and Kulkarni 1999a, 1999b). These partial agonist effects at D_1 and D_2 dopamine receptors would not be evident at high environmental temperatures and would not be anticipated to reduce antipsychotic drug–induced hyperthermia in the heat. However, partial agonism might be involved in reports of hypothermia associated with atypical antipsychotic drug treatment under cold ambient conditions (Parris et al. 2001; Phan et al. 1998). Furthermore, a protective effect in NMS cannot be excluded.

The major serotonin receptors implicated in the action of clozapine and other atypical antipsychotic agents include the following: $5\text{-}HT_{1A}$, $5\text{-}HT_{2A}$, $5\text{-}HT_{2C}$, $5\text{-}HT_3$, $5\text{-}HT_6$, and $5\text{-}HT_7$ (Meltzer 1999). As considered earlier, $5\text{-}HT_{1A}$ and $5\text{-}HT_{2C}$ receptors appear to be located "on-line" with dopamine receptors in the revised Bligh model's upper heat-loss pathway (Figure 2–5). Furthermore, $5\text{-}HT_{2A}$ receptors would probably function in that model's lower heat-production pathway. Several atypical antipsychotic drugs, including clozapine, quetiapine, and ziprasidone, are partial agonists at the $5\text{-}HT_{1A}$ receptor (Meltzer 1999). The presynaptic $5\text{-}HT_{1A}$ receptor is an autoreceptor located on cell bodies of the raphe neurons; stimulation leads to inhibition of the firing of serotonin neurons. Postsynaptic $5\text{-}HT_{1A}$ receptors are located in the terminal fields that receive serotoninergic innervation from the raphe nuclei; stimulation of these $5\text{-}HT_{1A}$ receptors leads to hyperpolarization of neurons—the opposite effect of stimulation of $5\text{-}HT_{2A}$ receptors. It is important to underscore the greater sensitivity of $5\text{-}HT_{1A}$ presynaptic autoreceptors compared with their postsynaptic counterparts (Millan 2000; Millan et al. 1998). Accordingly, partial agonists with intermediate efficacy (such as clozapine) preferentially activate $5\text{-}HT_{1A}$ autoreceptors while blocking their postsynaptic counterparts (Millan 2000). The serotonin system inhibits dopaminergic function at the level of the origin of the dopamine system in the midbrain as well as the terminal dopaminergic fields in the forebrain (Kapur and Remington 1996). By stimulating $5\text{-}HT_{1A}$ autoreceptors and, thus, inhibiting the firing of raphe serotonin neurons, atypical antipsychotics with $5\text{-}HT_{1A}$ partial agonist properties could increase neurotransmission in midbrain dopaminergic projections, yielding enhanced therapeutic efficacy. In contrast, by blocking postsynaptic $5\text{-}HT_{1A}$ receptors, which participate in serotonin-mediated thermoregulatory heat-loss mechanisms, atypical antipsychotics with 5-HT_{1A} partial agonism could contribute to hyperthermia in a hot environment (Figure 2–5).

Similar to dopamine receptors and postsynaptic 5-HT_{1A} receptors involved in thermoregulation, blockade of 5-HT_{2C} receptors would be anticipated to interrupt the revised Bligh model's upper heat-loss pathway and promote hyperthermia at high environmental temperatures (Figure 2–5). With the exception of quetiapine, each of the available atypical antipsychotics has moderate to high affinity for 5-HT_{2C} receptors (Weiden 2001). Additionally, several typical antipsychotic drugs, including chlorpromazine, thioridazine, and mesoridazine, have high affinities for 5-HT_{2C} receptors (B. Roth et al. 1999).

At present, substantial evidence supports the hypothesis that 5-HT_{2A} receptor blockade is critical for many of the therapeutic advantages of currently available atypical antipsychotic drugs (Meltzer et al. 1989). Clozapine, risperidone, olanzapine, quetiapine, and ziprasidone are all more potent 5-HT_{2A} than D_2 antagonists at appropriate doses (Meltzer 1999). As discussed previously, serotonin agonist–induced hyperthermia appears mediated by 5-HT_{2A} receptors that participate in the revised Bligh model's heat-production pathway (Figure 2–5). In the rat, 5-HT_{2A}-mediated hyperthermia is produced by an increase in metabolic rate and a decrease in skin temperature (Lin et al. 1998). Although not associated with hyperthermia, antipsychotic drug–induced 5-HT_{2A} receptor blockade could be involved in promoting hypothermia and could exert a protective effect against NMS.

In fact, two recent reports have described hypothermia occurring in patients treated with atypical antipsychotic drugs (Parris et al. 2001; Phan et al. 1998); 5-HT_2 receptor blockade was considered the primary pathogenetic mechanism. Our review would implicate the 5-HT_{2A} receptor subtype in particular. These cases differed from hypothermia cases reported during treatment with typical antipsychotic agents (Lazarus et al. 1989) in that cold exposure was not involved. Phan et al. (1998) postulated that their patient's hypothermic response, first to risperidone and then to olanzapine, had resulted from 5-HT_2 receptor blockade. Parris et al. (2001) reported single cases of hypothermia in association with olanzapine and quetiapine. They suggested that by antagonizing hypothalamic 5-HT_2 receptors, atypical antipsychotics most likely reduce the body's ability to adequately regulate internal temperature. Furthermore, they proposed that "antagonism of postsynaptic 5-HT_2 receptors may reduce the interaction between 5-HT and the receptor and cause an effective reduction in 5-HT," thus promoting hypothermia. As mentioned earlier in this chapter, some investigators have reported hypothermia during treatment with the 5-HT_{2A} receptor antagonists, such as ketanserin, alone (Cryan et al. 2000; Gudelsky et al.

1986), although others have failed to replicate this finding (Salmi and Ahlenius 1998).

Fever, Hyperthermia, and Heatstroke

In considering elevations in body temperature, it is important to note that the term *fever* refers to a discrete subtype of hyperthermia (Stitt 1979). Infections, inflammatory processes, mechanical trauma, neoplasms, immunological reactions, and other causes of tissue injury release various proteins, protein fragments, and bacterial lipopolysaccharide toxins that are collectively termed *exogenous pyrogens* (Schafer 1998). Exogenous pyrogens stimulate monocytes and macrophages to release cytokines such as interleukin-1, interleukin-6, and TNF-α, which are referred to as *endogenous pyrogens*. Endogenous pyrogens act on the hypothalamus to bring about an elevation in the set point, with a consequent increase in body temperature (Guyton and Hall 2000). This effect is thought to be mediated by local release of prostaglandins. Febrile hyperthermia is the product of coordinated effector responses requiring intact central thermoregulatory mechanisms. Other features of fever are 1) response to aspirin-like drugs, which are prostaglandin inhibitors; 2) lack of response to external cooling alone in the absence of aspirin-like agents (the body's tendency to defend the elevation in temperature dictated by the set point); and 3) the uncommon occurrence of fevers in excess of 41.1°C. As noted earlier, at least some cases of benign hyperthermia represent a drug fever—that is, fever resulting from an immunological reaction to the antipsychotic agent.

In contrast to fever, other types of hyperthermia involve either disordered central thermoregulation, impaired peripheral heat loss, excessive thermal challenge, or a combination of these factors (Clark and Lipton 1984; Lomax and Schonbaum 1998). Antipyretics are ineffective in nonfebrile hyperthermia because pyrogens and prostaglandins are not involved. Nonfebrile hyperthermia occurring independently of a hot environment may be the product of various hypermetabolic disorders such as thyrotoxicosis and pheochromocytoma; cerebral lesions affecting thermoregulatory centers, including tumors, infections, degenerative diseases, and vascular accidents; and withdrawal from ethanol, sedative-hypnotic drugs, or opiates. In addition, a wide variety of drugs may alter body temperature by acting on any component of the thermoregulatory system: thermosensors and their afferent pathways, thermoeffectors and their efferent pathways, and coordinating neurons within the CNS (including elevation of the set point) (Clark and Lipton 1984; Lomax and Schonbaum 1998).

Heatstroke is a life-threatening disorder requiring emergency medical

TABLE 2–1. Comparison of classic and exertional heatstroke

	Classic	Exertional
Age group affected	Elderly (or infants), men=women	Men, ages 15–45
State of health	Chronic illness common	Usually healthy
Activity	Sedentary	High activity level
Epidemic occurrence	Yes	No
Prevailing weather	Heat wave	Variable
Skin	Dry and hot	50% continue to sweat
Respiratory alkalosis	Dominant	Mild
Lactic acidosis	Absent or mild	Often marked
Rhabdomyolysis	Seldom severe	Severe
Creatine phosphokinase	Mildly elevated	Markedly elevated
Acute renal failure	<5% of patients	30% of patients
Disseminated intravascular coagulation	Mild	Marked
Hypocalcemia	Uncommon	Common
Hypoglycemia	Uncommon	Common
Irreversible central nervous system impairment	Elderly more susceptible	Less common

Source. Adapted from Knochel JP, Reed G: "Disorders of Heat Regulation," in *Maxwell and Kleeman's Clinical Disorders of Fluid and Electrolyte Metabolism.* Edited by Narins RG. New York, McGraw-Hill, 1994, pp. 1549–1590. Used with permission of McGraw-Hill Companies.

treatment. It is generally divided into two types: classic and exertional (Table 2–1). *Classic heatstroke* is characterized by body temperature above 40.6°C; anhidrosis; and profound CNS dysfunction with severe disorientation, delirium, or coma (Knochel and Reed 1994). Classic heatstroke typically occurs in epidemic fashion during summer heat waves when ambient temperatures frequently exceed 37.9°C or when lower ambient temperatures are accompanied by high relative humidity, and both temperature and humidity are sustained relentlessly through several days and nights (Knochel 1989; Knochel and Reed 1994). Thus, active perspiration is continuous but eventually fails, body temperature rises rapidly, and classic heatstroke supervenes. Most cases come to medical attention only after 3 or more days into the heat wave. Sudden collapse may occur independent of prodromal symptoms. Other patients may develop weakness, dizziness, nausea, and fainting spells up to 2 or 3 days before their collapse. Some victims may be found wandering about in a confusional state. Among those survivors who can recall, about half remember that sweating ceased before the onset of collapse (Knochel 1989). Some describe an associated sensation of coldness, accompanied by chills and gooseflesh. These manifestations probably indicate the onset of thermoregulatory failure and resemble the response to a pyrogen in which the body attempts to increase its temperature (Knochel and Reed 1994).

Older adults, the very young, or the infirm who are of lower socioeconomic status and live in large cities under conditions of low airflow (e.g., higher floors of multistory buildings) and a lack of air-conditioning are the most at risk for classic heatstroke. In one series associated with a severe heat wave, heatstroke rates were 10–12 times higher in persons age 65 years or older than in those younger than 65 and 3 times higher in African Americans than in whites (S.T. Jones et al. 1982). The age-adjusted heatstroke rates for men and woman were similar. However, men appear twice as likely to die from heat-related illness during a heat wave (National Center for Health Statistics 2000). In large cities, lack of airflow and the presence of heat release from streets and buildings prevent temperatures from falling during the night as they do in rural areas (Knochel 1989). If air-conditioning is available, such individuals may never develop acclimatization, leaving them vulnerable to heatstroke during "brownouts," or air-conditioning failure (Knochel and Reed 1994). Acclimatization to heat takes 2 weeks or more of exposure to heat and requires complex multisystem adaptations. The elderly are predisposed to classic heatstroke under such conditions on the basis of chronic illnesses, in particular cardiovascular, pulmonary, and renal disease; diabetes mellitus; and dementia; as well as decreased efficiency of sweating, impaired ability to acclimatize, and a tendency to be receiving medications that interfere with thermoregulation. Other risk factors in the general population include infectious illnesses, impaired sweat production (e.g., congenital absence of sweat glands, prickly heat, severe burns, scleroderma), obesity, various endocrinopathies, acute or chronic alcoholism, malnutrition, and chronic inactivity (Kilbourne et al. 1982; Knochel 1989).

In sharp contrast to the aged and debilitated patients typically involved in classic heatstroke, *exertional heatstroke* occurs primarily in young, healthy men with normal thermoregulatory capacity. In this instance, heat produced by muscular work in a hot environment exceeds the body's capacity to dissipate it. In the United States, the highest incidence of exertional heatstroke is found in marathon runners, less experienced football players, and military recruits (Knochel and Reed 1994). Overzealous training, requirements for performance that exceed human capacity, clothing that prevents vaporization of sweat (e.g., impervious plastic sweat clothing or leather football gear), and inadequate hydration and salt supplementation represent risk factors for the development of exertional heatstroke (Knochel 1989; Knochel and Reed 1994).

Unlike in classic heatstroke, about half of the patients with exertional heatstroke may continue to sweat in the acute phase. Furthermore, as sweat vaporizes, the skin may appear cool despite a high core body temperature. These factors may obscure the proper diagnosis and prevent prompt treatment. Although elevated levels of creatine phosphokinase (CPK) may be present in classic heatstroke, they rarely exceed 2,000 IU, and acute renal failure affects fewer than 5% of patients. In exertional heatstroke, massive muscle damage (rhabdomyolysis) is common, with marked CPK elevations (reported as high as 2,500,000 IU). Acute myoglobinuric renal failure is observed in 30% of patients with exertional heatstroke (Knochel and Reed 1994). Nearly all patients with classic heatstroke show respiratory alkalosis. In contrast, prominent lactic acidosis is often an early finding in exertional heatstroke and appears to have no bearing on the predicted outcome. However, lactic acidosis also may develop during extremely severe classic heatstroke complicated by heart failure or shock. In this form of heatstroke, lactic acidosis predicts an ominous outcome (Knochel 1989). Disseminated intravascular coagulation is often severe in exertional heatstroke but is less pronounced in classic heatstroke.

In general, patients with classic heatstroke show much less evidence of tissue damage than do young men with exertional heatstroke. Classic heatstroke patients with core temperatures as high as 43.7°C have been observed to recover without clear sequelae. In contrast, virtual total body destruction (somatolysis) has been seen during exertional heatstroke in young men whose core temperatures did not exceed 40.6°C (Knochel and Reed 1994). However, both forms of heatstroke may result in myocardial infarction and congestive heart failure, pancreatitis, hepatic failure, and adult respiratory distress syndrome. Mental status changes such as coma, stupor, and agitated delirium are common in both forms. CNS manifestations include grand mal seizures, pupillary abnormalities, and hemiplegia acutely, with cerebellar symptoms including ataxia and dysarthria a not infrequent permanent complication (Lefkowitz et al. 1983). Electron microscopic studies have detected alterations in the subcellular components of sweat glands, perhaps accounting for the observation that some survivors of heatstroke show a residual impairment in sweating accompanied by a persistent susceptibility to the effects of a hot environment (Knochel and Reed 1994).

Maintenance of muscle tone during heatstroke is variably described. Some researchers report that skeletal musculature is typically flaccid, with rigidity developing only following initiation of therapeutic cooling (Knochel 1989). Clark and Lipton (1984) stated that rigidity may develop secondary to hyperthermia during the later stages of heatstroke. Shibolet et al. (1976) noted that "profound rigidity with tonic contractions, coarse tremor, dystonic movement, and muscle cramps often alternate with a convulsive state" (p. 292) during heatstroke. However, increased muscle tone is almost never reported in cases of ADRHS (Bark 1982; Clark and Lipton 1984), in contrast to the muscular rigidity of NMS.

A variety of drugs have been associated with the development of heatstroke. Clark and Lipton (1984) stressed the value of dividing drug-related heatstroke into two broad categories: drug-facilitated heatstroke and drug-induced heatstroke. In *drug-facilitated heatstroke*, direct effects of drugs on the thermoregulatory system impair its capacity to increase heat loss in response to an imposed heat load. Agents exert only a permissive influence that favors heat storage; the development of hyperthermia hinges on exposure to a hot environment or heat production during strenuous exercise. Antipsychotic drugs and anticholinergic agents represent two categories of drugs that, at therapeutic dosages, are frequently implicated in drug-facilitated heatstroke. Anticholinergics inhibit sweating, whereas antipsychotics interfere with central thermoregulation. In addition, antipsychotic drugs themselves possess varying degrees of peripheral anticholinergic activity, which may further facilitate heatstroke.

Agents involved in *drug-induced heatstroke* increase endogenous heat production and cause hyperthermia independent of environmental conditions. Drugs may act directly on peripheral effector mechanisms for heat production (e.g., increased cellular metabolism associated with salicylate intoxication and anesthetic effects on muscle in malignant hyperthermia). Drugs may act directly on the CNS to cause heatstroke, as in intoxication with anticholinergics (atropine poisoning vs. anticholinergic treatment at therapeutic dosages); amphetamines and derivatives, such as fenfluramine and 3,4-methylenedioxymethamphetamine (MDMA) or "Ecstasy"; cocaine; heterocyclic antidepressants; monoamine oxidase inhibitors; lysergic acid diethylamide (LSD); phencyclidine (PCP); marijuana; xanthine derivatives; and others. Pathophysiological mechanisms by which drugs acting directly on the CNS may induce heatstroke are reviewed in detail in Chapter 4. Included are mechanisms for increased psychomotor activity, enhanced muscle tone, constriction of cutaneous vasculature, and direct drug effects on the hypothalamus. The involvement of serotoninergic agents in drug-induced heatstroke is further considered in Chapter 3.

Antipsychotic drugs clearly exert actions on the hypothalamic thermoregulatory mechanisms. Their suppression of central heat loss pathways appears to be involved in the pathogenesis of both ADRHS and NMS. However, in NMS, excess heat seems to derive primarily from hypermetabolism of skeletal muscle caused by antipsychotic drug–induced extrapyramidal rigidity and possibly from direct effects of antipsychotics on skeletal muscle (Caroff et al. 2001c; Mann et al. 2000). Thus, NMS represents a genuine drug-induced heatstroke. In contrast, ADRHS is best viewed as drug-facilitated heatstroke in which antipsychotics simply increase vulnerability to a well-described form of environmental heat illness by interfering with heat dissipation.

🗿 Psychiatric Aspects of Heatstroke

Risk Factors

The high prevalence in psychiatric patients of factors that predispose to both classic and exertional heatstroke places this population at particular risk (Bark 1982, 1998; Lazarus 1985a; Mann and Boger 1978; Wise 1973). In the wake of deinstitutionalization, increasing numbers of homeless patients have been exposed to high environmental temperature and humidity during heat waves. Such patients often wear multiple layers of clothing, severely compromising evaporative heat loss. It is possible that certain psychiatric patients do not perceive an excessively hot environment as noxious and thus fail to remove themselves from it (Bark 1998). In addition, psychiatric patients tend to live in small, crowded rooms with poor ventilation or no air-conditioning, often on the higher floors of multistory buildings, conditions discussed previously as predisposing to heatstroke. Poor nutrition or delusional beliefs concerning nutrition (e.g., food being poisoned) may lead to inadequate fluid and salt intake necessary for evaporative heat loss.

Hospitalized psychiatric patients are also at increased risk for heatstroke. Some psychiatric inpatient units may not be air-conditioned. Seclusion rooms represent a specific concern, as they may be small, be hot, and lack cross-ventilation. Increased motor activity associated with agitation, struggling against restraints, and psychotic excitement clearly increase the likelihood of exertional heatstroke. The more frequent occurrence of such behaviors in male patients may in part explain Bark's (1982) observation that ADRHS affected 9 males to every 1 female and that the sex ratio of patients who died was 21 males to 1 female.

Recently, we have been consulted about several cases in which psychotic patients were successfully treated in the hospital during the summer, only to die unexpectedly from heatstroke within days after discharge (Caroff et al. 2000b). These cases indicated to us that the time immediately after discharge from an extended hospital stay might represent an important but neglected high-risk period for heatstroke. Patients may be more vulnerable to heatstroke after discharge for several reasons. First, patients who have been noncompliant with their medications before admission have a significantly reduced ability to dissipate heat once antipsychotic and anticholinergic medications are reinstituted during hospitalization. Second, after recovery, patients may feel more energetic and attempt to compensate for activities they missed while hospitalized, predisposing to exertional heatstroke. Many clinicians and patients may be unaware of how little physical activity it takes to raise body temperatures to life-threatening levels in a hot, humid environment when heat-loss mechanisms are impaired by drugs. Third, patients who have been sedentary in an air-conditioned hospital environment are neither physically conditioned nor acclimatized to the heat. Finally, resumption of drug or alcohol use after discharge further increases the risk of heatstroke on discharge during a heat wave.

Before the introduction of antipsychotics, it was suggested that psychiatric patients are at increased risk for heatstroke, perhaps because the neurotransmitters involved in thermoregulation also participate in the disease processes of schizophrenia and mood disorders (Bark 1998). Finkelman and Stephens (1936) and Gottlieb and Linder (1935) presented data suggesting that, compared with nonschizophrenic individuals, schizophrenic patients develop relative hypothermia in the cold and hyperthermia in the heat (i.e., poikilothermia). Curiously, antipsychotic drugs appear to exert this same effect on both human and animal thermoregulation. Recently, Hermesh et al. (2000) subjected schizophrenic patients to a heat challenge and found that they had impaired heat tolerance compared with healthy control subjects. Noting that these results were consistent with studies of thermoregulatory dysfunction in antipsychotic drug–treated animals, they concluded that it was unclear if this hyperthermic response reflected a dysfunction associated with schizophrenia, an antipsychotic drug–induced effect, or both (Hermesh et al. 2000).

Role of Antipsychotic Drugs

In 1956, Ayd reported a case of fatal heatstroke in a 41-year-old chlorpromazine-treated schizophrenic patient exposed to hot weather. He discussed evidence that chlorpromazine could impair hypothalamic thermoregulatory mechanisms. He postulated that death in this case was the result of chlorpromazine's effects on the hypothalamus "accentuated by the high environmental temperature" (p. 191).

Zelman and Guillan (1970) reported three similar cases occurring during a heat wave, noting a regrettable lack of reference to ADRHS in journals, textbooks, and product information summaries. These authors cited the findings of Kollias and Bullard (1964) that phenothiazine-induced suppression of hypothalamic thermoregulation renders rats thermally dependent on their environment, leading to hyperthermia in the heat. Case reports of ADRHS suggested a similar pattern of antipsychotic drug–induced thermal dependency in humans.

Subsequent to Zelman and Guillan's (1970) article, ADRHS became more frequently reported, particularly in the context of its delimitation from NMS (Caroff 1980; Lazarus 1985a; Mann and Boger 1978). Bark (1982) reviewed 48 cases of heatstroke occurring in patients taking typical antipsychotic drugs. Their mean age of 44 was surprising considering that heatstroke occurring in the general population usually involves persons older than 65. In 43 patients, hyperthermia was viewed as the product of antipsychotic drug–induced suppression of heat-loss mechanisms in the heat. The remaining five cases, however, did not involve high environmental temperatures. Instead, hyperthermia was attributed to exercise, hyperactivity, agitation during sedative-hypnotic withdrawal, and agitation with impaired heat dissipation during sheet restraint.

Clark and Lipton (1984) reviewed 45 cases of ADRHS related to treatment with typical antipsychotics and involving a maximal body temperature of at least 40°C. Most of these cases also had been reviewed in Bark's (1982) series. Clark and Lipton (1984) concluded that among drug-related hyperthermias, ADRHS most closely mimics classic heatstroke rather than exertional heatstroke in phenomenology and pathophysiology. Of the 45 patients, only 6 had maximal body temperature elevations below 41.1°C, 16 had maximal body temperatures between 41.1°C and 42.1°C, and 23 had temperatures above 42.1°C. Mortality figures for these three groups—0%, 38%, and 61%, respectively—paralleled those of classic heatstroke, with higher temperatures associated with increasing degrees of multisystem damage and an unfavorable prognosis. This contrasted with findings in NMS as reviewed by Clark and Lipton (1984), in which body temperature exceeded 40°C in only half of the patients and 41.1°C in fewer than 20% of the patients. Furthermore, mortality rates across various temperature ranges in NMS were similar, suggesting that the extent of elevation in body temperature itself is seldom the major factor accounting for death in NMS.

Both Bark (1982) and Clark and Lipton (1984) noted that in the absence of concurrent treatment with anticholinergic antiparkinsonian agents or heterocyclic antidepressants, antipsychotic drugs involved in causing ADRHS were more commonly those with greater degrees of peripheral anticholinergic activity, such as phenothiazines of the alkylamino group (chlorpromazine and promazine) and the piperidine group (thioridazine and mepazine). In fact, mepazine, the most potent anticholinergic of all antipsychotics, was withdrawn from use because of case reports of heatstroke (Bark 1998). Cases of ADRHS attributed to high-potency agents such as the piperazine phenothiazines (perphenazine, trifluoperazine, and fluphenazine), the thioxanthene antipsychotic thiothixene, and the butyrophenone antipsychotic haloperidol—all low in anticholinergic activity (Mann et al. 1999)—involved concomitant treatment with anticholinergic agents in all but three reported cases: single cases associated with trifluoperazine, fluphenazine, and haloperidol. These findings suggest that the anticholinergic-induced inhibition of sweating contributed to the development of ADRHS in most instances. Still, those few reports of ADRHS in patients treated solely with high-potency agents suggest that antipsychotics must be regarded as capable of causing ADRHS independent of adjunctive therapy with anticholinergic agents or the intrinsic anticholinergic effects exerted by antipsychotics themselves.

Following a comprehensive review of the literature, we were unable to identify any clear cases of ADRHS secondary to atypical antipsychotic drugs. This was surprising in view of the ability of atypical antipsychotics to attenuate D_2 agonist–induced hypothermia (Oerther and Ahlenius 2000). Furthermore, it is clear that NMS can result from treatment with atypical antipsychotics and that it often presents with the classic features and course of illness reported previously in association with typical antipsychotic drugs (see Chapter 1). Consistent with the dopamine receptor blockade hypothesis of NMS, this suggested that NMS hyperthermia can be triggered by drug-induced D_2 receptor occupancy lower than that associated with common extrapyramidal side effects and perhaps lower than that required for therapeutic antipsychotic efficacy (Caroff et al. 2000a). As considered previously, there are distinct differences in the pathogenetic mechanisms accounting for hyperthermia in ADRHS and NMS. Antipsychotic drug–induced dopamine receptor blockade impairs heat loss in both conditions. In NMS, however, by inducing extrapyramidal rigidity, it also represents the primary mechanism for excessive heat production. As such, dopamine receptor antagonism plays a broader role in the etiology of NMS compared with ADRHS, and lesser degrees of dopamine receptor occupancy might be adequate to precipitate symptoms in the former condition.

Still, when considering the differential actions of atypical antipsychotics and typical agents on selected serotonin receptor subtypes, their overall effect would appear to predispose to ADRHS. Both 5-HT_{2C} and postsynaptic 5-HT_{1A} receptors participate in serotonin-mediated thermoregulatory heat-loss mechanisms, and their blockade by atypical agents with 5-HT_{2C} antagonism or partial 5-HT_{1A} agonism (antagonists at postsynaptic 5-HT_{1A} receptors) would be expected to promote hyperthermia in a hot environment. Furthermore, both clozapine and olanzapine possess considerable anticholinergic activity, which could predispose to heatstroke. In recent years, our combined clinical experience and work involving the Neuroleptic Malignant Syndrome Information Service database has suggested that cases of ADRHS are often misidentified as NMS. This seems to be true of a recent report of hyperthermia occurring in a bipolar patient treated with risperidone 6 mg/day, thioridazine 25 mg/day, and lithium 500 mg/day (McGugan 2001). It appears to us that the relative risk of ADRHS occurring in association with the use of atypical versus typical antipsychotics remains unclear. As atypical antipsychotics become more widely used as first-line agents in the treatment of psychosis, more broad-based, prospective data on ADRHS with these drugs may become available. In fact, a recent consultation to the Neuroleptic Malignant Syndrome Information Service telephone hotline appears to represent ADHRS of the exertional type occurring during combined treatment with quetiapine, ziprasidone, and diphenhydramine.

Clinical Vignette

A 43-year-old man with a long history of schizophrenia developed diabetes mellitus while taking olanzapine and was switched to quetiapine 400 mg/day. He did well for several months until mid-summer, when he began to have insomnia, restlessness, auditory hallucinations, and ritualistic behavior. Quetiapine was increased to 500 mg/day, and diphenhydramine 50 mg at bedtime was started for insomnia. A week later, his psychiatric condition had deteriorated, and he presented as restless and sweating. Ambient temperature was described as "hot," and the patient was noted to be drinking large amounts of iced tea. Quetiapine was decreased to 400 mg/day, and ziprasidone 40 mg/day was started. Three days later, he was observed to be "stooped and pacing." The next day, he suddenly collapsed outdoors and became unresponsive. On admission to the emergency department, his rectal temperature was reported as 42.2°C. The presence of muscle rigidity or tremor was considered questionable. However, his eyes and head deviated to the left. Results from brain computed tomography and cerebrospinal fluid analysis were unremarkable. CPK was reported as 91,000 IU. He developed acute renal failure requiring dialysis. He awakened confused, delusional, and hallucinating.

The abrupt onset of this episode, its occurrence in the context of agitated behavior during hot summer weather, and the absence of significant muscle rigidity favor a diagnosis of exertional ADRHS over NMS in this case. As discussed earlier, about half of patients with exertional heatstroke continue to sweat during the acute phase. Heatstroke appears to have been facilitated by therapeutic dosages of quetiapine, ziprasidone, and diphenhydramine.

🗿 Treatment and Prevention

ADRHS is a preventable condition. Bark (1998) reported that prior to 1979, patients hospitalized in state psychiatric hospitals in the New York

City area had twice the relative risk of dying during a heat wave compared with the general population. However, the risk was clearly reduced after preventive measures, including installation of air-conditioning, close monitoring of medications, and staff training in prevention and recognition of heatstroke, were instituted. All persons involved in the treatment, care, and supervision of psychiatric patients should be aware of the signs and symptoms of heatstroke and the need for immediate action. A comprehensive discussion of the treatment of heatstroke is beyond the scope of this chapter; the interested reader is referred to reviews elsewhere (Khosla and Guntupalli 1999; Knochel 1989; Knochel and Reed 1994).

All forms of treatment aim at rapid cooling, fluid and electrolyte support, and management of seizures. In some cases, removing the patient from sunlight, removing the patient's clothing, wetting the body, and fanning to promote vaporization will be sufficient. However, most patients require intensive therapy, best rendered by a coordinated team in an emergency department setting. Emergency departments in high-risk areas should have the potential to convert space into a "heatstroke room" with tubs, floor drains, and other special equipment necessary for the rapid management of heatstroke patients (R.J. Anderson et al. 1983).

During summer heat waves, psychiatric patients must be warned to avoid excessive heat and sunlight exposure, discouraged from performing vigorous exercise or physical labor, and urged to drink adequate amounts of fluid. Air-conditioning probably represents the most effective means of preventing heatstroke; even an hour a day in the supermarket is helpful (Bark 1998). A primary consideration in minimizing the risk of heatstroke should be the administration of antipsychotic drugs at the lowest possible dosages. In Bark's (1998) sample of hospitalized psychiatric patients, the risk of death during heat waves initially decreased following the introduction of antipsychotic drugs but rose to its highest level in the late 1970s, when higher antipsychotic dosages were routinely used. In the treatment of acute psychoses, rapid tranquilization and "megadose" techniques, now increasingly out of vogue, if used at all, should be used with particular caution during hot summer days. Benzodiazepines, rather than antipsychotics, should be selected for treatment of agitation, and anticholinergics should be kept to a minimum (Bark 1998). In keeping with their role as a facilitator rather than a direct cause of heatstroke, antipsychotic drugs can generally be restarted following ADRHS, with little concern about recurrence of heatstroke in the absence of high environmental temperature or excessive endogenous heat production. This differs from the very real risk of recurrence on antipsychotic drug rechallenge in patients recovered from an NMS episode, especially if rechallenge is undertaken prematurely.

🗿 Conclusion

Numerous clinical case reports involving patients treated with typical antipsychotic drugs and exposed to extremes of thermal challenge indicate that these agents can significantly impair thermoregulation. A consistent observation has been the tendency of typical antipsychotic drugs to render patients thermally dependent on their environment, leading to hyperthermia in the heat. Similar findings have been reported in animal experiments across a wide variety of species. In the absence of human research data, animal studies form the basis for understanding the effects of antipsychotic drugs on thermoregulation. This literature indicates that antipsychotics impair central thermoregulation in the PO/AH and other areas and that this impairment appears to be mediated primarily through effects on CNS monoamine systems.

In view of evidence supporting a prominent role for dopamine in hypothalamic thermoregulatory mechanisms, all antipsychotics, whether typical or atypical, could impair heat loss by antagonizing D_2 as well as D_1 and D_3 dopamine receptors. Furthermore, both 5-HT_{2C} and postsynaptic 5-HT_{1A} receptors participate in serotonin-mediated heat-loss mechanisms, and their blockade by atypical antipsychotics with 5-HT_{2C} antagonism or partial 5-HT_{1A} agonism could further promote hyperthermia in a hot environment. Although 5-HT_{2A} receptors participate in the revised Bligh model's heat-production pathway, and their blockade would be associated with hyperthermia, 5-HT_{2A} antagonism might be implicated in hypothermia during atypical antipsychotic drug treatment and could provide a protective effect against NMS. Furthermore, clozapine's partial agonist properties at D_1 and D_2 receptors could predispose toward hypothermia in the cold and, conceivably, attenuate the hyperthermia of NMS under such conditions, as could the D_2 partial agonism of olanzapine.

Suppression of central heat-loss mechanisms by antipsychotics appears to be involved in the pathogenesis of both ADRHS and NMS. However, in NMS, excess heat appears to be derived primarily from antipsychotic drug–induced extrapyramidal rigidity and possibly from direct effects of antipsychotics on skeletal muscle. In ADRHS, excess heat comes from a hot environment. Thus, NMS appears to represent a genuine form of drug-induced heatstroke. In contrast, ADRHS is best viewed as a drug-facilitated heatstroke in which antipsychotics increase vulnerability to a well-described form of environmental heat illness by interfering with heat dissipation. Further, most ADRHS cases more closely mimic classic rather than exertional heatstroke in phenomenology and pathophysiology. It appears likely that the anticholinergic effects of antipsychotics themselves, or anticholinergic agents often administered concurrently with typical antipsychotics, can facilitate ADRHS. However, high-potency typical anti-psychotics with little anticholinergic activity appear capable of causing ADRHS when they are administered alone. Although the risk of ADRHS occurring in association with atypical antipsychotic drugs remains unclear, it is unlikely to prove negligible.

C H A P T E R   3

Serotonin Syndrome

The development of medications with relatively selective effects on serotonin neurotransmission or specific effects on serotonin receptor subtypes greatly expanded the therapeutic arsenal for a variety of psychiatric, neurological, and medical illnesses (Keck and Arnold 2000). Selective serotonin reuptake inhibitors (SSRIs) are among the most commonly prescribed medications in the United States. The success of these agents has been due, in part, to their superior safety profile in comparison with older agents that were associated with unwanted, nonselective effects on other neurotransmitter systems (e.g., histaminergic, cholinergic, and α_1-adrenergic receptor antagonism). Because of their selective effects on serotoninergic neurotransmission, the side effects of SSRIs are usually the result of serotoninergic activity in nontarget organ systems or neuronal pathways. Recently, at least two SSRIs—paroxetine and sertraline (Amsterdam 1998)—have been shown to have significant reuptake inhibition of norepinephrine and dopamine, respectively. Nevertheless, one of the most severe adverse events associated with serotoninergic agents—the *serotonin syndrome*—appears to be mediated primarily by excessive serotoninergic activity.

The serotonin syndrome is an uncommon but potentially fatal complication of treatment with serotoninergic agents. This syndrome is distinguished from more common side effects of these agents by the severity, duration, and co-occurrence of a constellation of specific serotoninergically mediated systemic and central nervous system (CNS) effects (Lane and Baldwin 1997). In the last decade, coincident with the expanding use of serotoninergic medications, numerous cases of the serotonin syndrome

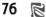

have been reported in the literature. In addition, preliminary studies have begun to estimate its incidence, identify risk factors, suggest treatment approaches, and formulate more reliable operational criteria to define the syndrome. Given these advances and the potential seriousness of the serotonin syndrome, it is increasingly important for physicians to be familiar with its clinical features, pathogenesis, and treatment.

Historical Background

The first reports of the serotonin syndrome appeared in the 1950s, coincident with the beginning of the modern era of psychopharmacology and, in particular, with the development of monoamine oxidase inhibitors (MAOIs) for the treatment of depression, hypertension, and tuberculosis (Mitchell 1955; Pare and Sandler 1959). The first report used the term *toxic encephalitis* to describe a patient's syndrome that consisted of mental status changes, myoclonus, ankle clonus, and Babinski's reflexes while receiving meperidine and the MAOI iproniazid (Mitchell 1955). The significance of this adverse drug interaction was not immediately recognized. In the early 1960s, the effects of the serotonin precursor L-tryptophan on the CNS became the focus of intensive study (Mills 1997). As part of this research, Oates and Sjoerdsma (1960) described the "indolamine syndrome" in several patients with hypertension who received single doses of L-tryptophan (20–50 mg) during treatment with the MAOI β-phenylisopropylhydrazine.

The features of indolamine syndrome included altered mental status, restlessness, diaphoresis, myoclonus, ataxia, and hyperreflexia. However, no significant changes in vital signs were observed. These investigators were the first to specifically propose that elevations in serotonin and tryptamine were responsible for this clinical syndrome. Other reports also appeared that suggested the role of CNS serotoninergic activity in mediating a syndrome characterized by behavioral, autonomic, and neuromuscular abnormalities. B. Smith and Prockop (1962) described a syndrome of euphoria, hyperreflexia, ankle clonus, and sustained nystagmus in healthy volunteers following administration of high doses (70 and 90 mg/kg) of L-tryptophan. These findings paralleled similar observations in rhesus monkeys induced by high doses of L-tryptophan (Curzon et al. 1963). A steady progression of clinical reports describing adverse drug interactions involving not only MAOIs and meperidine (Denton et al. 1962; Vigran 1964) but also MAOIs and tricyclics (F. Ayd 1961; Beaumont 1973; Grantham et al. 1964) appeared over the subsequent two decades. Notably, in addition to mental status and neuromuscular abnormalities, hyperthermia and autonomic nervous system instability were reported as a consequence of these interactions.

Insel et al. (1982) first introduced the term *serotonin syndrome* in the scientific literature. Sternbach (1991) conducted the first comprehensive clinical review, which summarized 12 clinical reports involving 38 patients. The publication of this review, along with the increasingly widespread use of serotoninergic medications, heightened clinical awareness of and stimulated research interest in the syndrome. For example, 133 reports involving 168 patients with suspected serotonin syndrome have been published since Sternbach's (1991) review. Thus, the history of scientific interest in the serotonin syndrome in many ways resembles that of neuroleptic malignant syndrome (NMS), with a heightened awareness following the publication of the first scholarly review (Caroff 1980).

🗝 Incidence

There is no estimate of the incidence of the serotonin syndrome. This is not surprising because its incidence is likely to be dependent on the criteria used to define the syndrome, specific medications and combinations of medications, pharmacokinetics, dose, and drug interactions. For example, as described later in this chapter, the risk of the serotonin syndrome is likely to be substantially higher in patients receiving MAOIs in combination with other medications that enhance serotoninergic neurotransmission.

To date, seven studies have estimated the incidence of the serotonin syndrome in association with specific medications or combinations of medications (Ebert et al. 1997; Hegerl et al. 1998; Kudo et al. 1997; Lejoyeux et al. 1993; MacKay et al. 1999; Richard et al. 1997; A.L. Weiner 1999). In the first clinical epidemiological study, Lejoyeux et al. (1993) assessed 38 inpatients with major depression treated for 4 weeks with clomipramine in naturalistic conditions for signs and symptoms of the syndrome as defined by criteria proposed by Sternbach (1991). All prior psychotropic medications were discontinued for 1 week before clomipramine was begun, and patients who received antipsychotics, fluoxetine, or MAOIs within 6 weeks of clomipramine administration were excluded. Ten (26.3%) of the 38 patients met criteria for serotonin syndrome, displaying tremor, diaphoresis, shivering, and myoclonus. Two other patients discontinued clomipramine because of generalized tremor and severe myoclonus, respectively. Although 32% of the patients were affected, 88% of the symptoms were transient, lasting less than 1 week, and abated without treatment interruption. These data suggested that when broadly defined, symptoms of serotonin syndrome were common in patients receiving clomipramine but were most often transient and usually did not alter treatment. The findings of this first study were limited by the unblinded assessments and lack of a control group.

In the second survey, Kudo et al. (1997) also estimated the incidence of the syndrome in 66 inpatients with major depression treated with clomipramine monotherapy. The primary aim of the study was to compare two sets of diagnostic criteria (discussed in detail later in this chapter) in estimating the incidence of serotonin syndrome. When Sternbach's (1991) criteria were applied, 8 (12.1%) patients developed signs and symptoms consistent with serotonin syndrome, whereas only 2 (3.0%) met the more restrictive criteria of Dursun et al. (1995).

In the third survey, Richard et al. (1997) asked 63 investigators participating in the Parkinson Study Group to estimate the frequency of serotonin syndrome in patients with Parkinson's disease treated with the combination of the MAOI selegiline and another antidepressant. Investigators responded to a questionnaire; for suspected cases, more detailed data were requested. Respondents (75% of the sample polled) estimated that approximately 4,565 patients received the combination of selegiline and an antidepressant. Of these patients, 11 (0.24%) were considered to have characteristics consistent with serotonin syndrome, and only 2 (0.04%) were considered serious. In addition, no patients met Sternbach's (1991) criteria for serotonin syndrome. The survey method used by these investigators is vulnerable to underdiagnosis and underreporting by respondents and a lack of standardization of assessment for the syndrome. In addition, the estimates are applicable only to the particular combination of selegiline with other antidepressants.

Ebert et al. (1997) prospectively assessed 200 consecutive patients treated with fluvoxamine (mean dose=200 mg/day) for serotonin syndrome by Sternbach's (1991) criteria. In this naturalistic study, 91 (45.5%) patients received other psychotropic medications, including tricyclics, reversible MAOIs, lithium, buspirone, or opiates. Over a cumulative 8,200 days of treatment exposure, no patients had "full-blown" serotonin syndrome. Three (1.5%) patients experienced mental status changes, insomnia, agitation, confusion, and incoherent thoughts without other signs or symptoms of the syndrome. This study was limited by the lack of a control group and unblinded assessments.

Hegerl et al. (1998) modified Sternbach's (1991) criteria to develop the Serotonin Syndrome Scale (SSS) to formally rate the severity of the syndrome. In the first study of the scale's validity (discussed in greater detail later in this chapter in the "Diagnosis" section), 5 (11.9%) of 42 patients receiving paroxetine in combination with other serotoninergic agents exceeded the minimum threshold criteria for the syndrome.

A.L. Weiner (1999) conducted a retrospective review of emergency department records of patients who received a single dose of meperidine during emergency department visits. During a 1-year period, 26 (9.9%) of

262 patients who received meperidine also were receiving serotoninergic agents (SSRIs, $n=15$; other antidepressants, $n=11$; lithium, $n=4$; tramadol, $n=3$; phentermine, $n=2$; fenfluramine, $n=2$). No signs or symptoms of serotonin syndrome were documented for any of these patients. However, the results of this survey were limited by its retrospective approach, reliance on patient report of concomitant medications, potential underestimation because of underreporting or recording of signs and symptoms in mild cases, and lack of follow-up beyond the acute treatment period in the emergency department.

In the most recent study, MacKay et al. (1999) conducted a postmarketing surveillance survey of 11,834 patients treated with nefazodone in England. Patients were systematically identified by means of prescription data from 1996 to 1997. Questionnaires were sent to prescribing general practitioners 6 months after the date of the first nefazodone prescription. Fifty-three patients with two or more of Sternbach's criteria for serotonin syndrome were followed up. Incidence rates were calculated and expressed as number of patients per 1,000 patient-months of treatment. Of the 53 patients, 19 (0.4 cases per 1,000) met criteria for the syndrome. Seven received nefazodone alone, four received nefazodone with benzodiazepines, one received nefazodone with valproate, one received nefazodone with lithium, and one received nefazodone with dothiepin. The investigators also reported incidence rates of patients who met two or more of Sternbach's criteria for serotonin syndrome with other serotoninergic agents from postmarketing surveillance data. These incidence rate estimates per 1,000 patient-months of treatment were fluoxetine 0.5, sertraline 0.6, paroxetine 0.9, moclobemide 0.5, and venlafaxine 0.9. Although these are the first population-based data regarding the incidence of serotonin syndrome, the survey method is vulnerable to the quality of physician reporting. Nevertheless, MacKay et al. (1999) had a remarkable 96.2% questionnaire return rate. Equally remarkably, 85.4% of the respondents were unaware of the serotonin syndrome.

The available surveys have significant methodological limitations. A blinded, prospective, naturalistic survey with patients not receiving nonserotoninergic agents as control subjects is needed to better define the incidence of serotonin syndrome in a large clinical population. The results of the surveys to date suggest that serotonin syndrome is a relatively uncommon complication of treatment with serotoninergic agents. The most important risk for developing the syndrome, as reviewed later, may lie in specific medications and combinations of medications that appear to account for a greater proportion of cases described in the literature and for particularly severe and lethal manifestations of the syndrome.

🗐 Onset and Predisposing Factors

Serotoninergic Medications

Nearly all medications that enhance CNS serotoninergic neurotransmission have been reported in association with cases of the serotonin syndrome (Table 3–1). Since the cases reviewed by Sternbach (1991), the most commonly implicated agents reported in subsequent case reports and case series have been combinations of MAOIs (reversible and irreversible) and tricyclics (N=18) (Brodribb et al. 1995; Chan et al. 1998; Corkeron 1995; Dardennes et al. 1998; Ferrer-Dufol et al. 1998; Francois et al. 1997; Gillman 1995, 1996, 1997b; Hernandez et al. 1995; Hoes and Zeijpveld 1996; Jahr et al. 1994; Kuisma 1995; Neuvonen et al. 1993; Nierenberg and Semprebon 1993; Spigset et al. 1993) and MAOIs and SRIs (N=34) (Brannan et al. 1994; Brubacher et al. 1996; Chan et al. 1998; Coplan and Gorman 1993; Diamond et al. 1998; Dingemanse et al. 1998; FitzSimmons and Metha 1999; Graber et al. 1994; Graudins et al. 1998; Heisler et al. 1996; Hilton et al. 1997; Hodgman et al. 1997; Keltner and Harris 1994; Kirrane et al. 1995; Lappin and Auchincloss 1994; Miller et al. 1991; Neuvonen et al. 1993; Ooi 1995; Phillips and Ringo 1995; Power et al. 1995; Roxanas and Machado 1998; L.A. Weiner et al. 1998). These combinations also have been involved in 11 (61.1%) of the 18 fatal cases of serotonin syndrome. Serotonin syndrome has been reported when an MAOI was used in combination with L-tryptophan (Price et al. 1992), dextromethorphan (Hoes and Zeijpveld 1996; Nierenberg and Semprebon 1993), or clonazepam (Butzkueven 1997). Tricyclics combined with alprazolam (Cano-Munoz et al. 1995), amoxapine (Nisijima 2000), clonazepam (Rosebush et al. 1999), SRIs (Alderman and Lee 1996; Brooks 1998; Molaie 1997; Perry 2000), lithium (Kojima et al. 1993), SRIs and lithium (Muly et al. 1993; Sobanski et al. 1997), trazodone and lithium (Nisijima et al. 1996), nefazodone and thioridazine (Chan et al. 1998), and *m*-chlorophenylpiperazine (m-CPP) (Price et al. 1992) also have been associated with the syndrome. SSRIs in combination with lithium (Ohman and Spigset 1993), venlafaxine (Bhatara et al. 1998; Chan et al. 1998; Gitlin 1997), buspirone (Baetz and Malcolm 1995; Spigset and Adielsson 1997), dextromethorphan (Chan et al. 1998; Skop et al. 1994; Zimmerschied and Harry 1998), carbamazepine (Dursun et al. 1993), clonazepam (Rella and Hoffman 1998), mirtazapine (Benazzi 1997), m-CPP (Klaassen et al. 1998), nefazodone (John et al. 1997), trazodone (George and Godleski 1996; R.R. Reeves and Bullen 1995), risperidone (Hamilton and Malone 2000), sumatriptan (Gardner and Lynd 1998; Mathew et al. 1996), dihydroergotamine (Mathew et al. 1996), and tramadol (Egberts et al. 1997; Kesavan and Sobala 1999; Lantz et al. 1998; B.J. Mason and Blackburn 1997) have been reported to produce

TABLE 3–1. Drugs potentiating serotonin in the central nervous system

Inhibition of serotonin reuptake
Amitriptyline
Bromocriptine
Citalopram
Clomipramine
Desipramine
Dextromethorphan
Fenfluramine
Fluoxetine
Fluvoxamine
Imipramine
Meperidine
Mirtazapine
Nefazodone
Nortriptyline
Paroxetine
Pethidine
Sertraline
Tramadol
Trazodone
Venlafaxine

Inhibition of serotonin catabolism
Isocarboxazid
Moclobemide
Phenelzine
Selegiline
Tranylcypromine

Enhancement of serotonin release
Amphetamines
Cocaine
Dextromethorphan
Fenfluramine
Meperidine
3,4-Methylenedioxymethamphetamine (MDMA)
Sibutramine

Serotonin agonists
Buspirone
Dihydroergotamine
Lithium
m-Chlorophenylpiperazine (m-CPP)
Sumatriptan
Trazodone

Enhancement of serotonin synthesis
L-Tryptophan

Source. Adapted from Keck PE Jr, Arnold LM: "Serotonin Syndrome." *Psychiatric Annals* 30:333–343, 2000. Used with permission.

serotonin syndrome. Combinations of nefazodone with trazodone (Margolese and Chouinard 2000), fluoxetine (D.L. Smith and Wenegrat 2000), valproate, and dothiepin (MacKay et al. 1999) have been reported in association with the syndrome. Similarly, serotonin syndrome has been reported with trazodone alone (R. Rao 1997) and a combination of trazodone and buspirone (Goldberg and Huk 1992). The syndrome also has been described in association with venlafaxine overdose (Coorey and Wenck 1998; Daniels 1998; Graudins et al. 1998) and when venlafaxine was combined with lithium (Mekler and Woggon 1997). Other cases have been associated with monotherapy with SRIs (Bastani et al. 1996; Graudins et al. 1998; Hegerl et al. 1998; Lenzi et al. 1993; MacKay et al. 1999; Pao and Tipnis 1997), clomipramine (Kudo et al. 1997; Lejoyeux et al. 1992), moclobemide (Fischer 1995), m-CPP (Klaassen ct al. 1998), and sumatriptan (Mathew et al. 1996). Of nontherapeutic agents, 3,4-methylenedioxymethamphetamine (MDMA or "Ecstasy") has been implicated in at least 14 reports involving 14 patients (Bedford Russell et al. 1992; C. Brown and Osterloh 1987; Campkin and Davies 1992; Chadwick et al. 1991; Demirkiran et al. 1996; Denborough and Hopkinson 1997; Gillman 1997a; Logan et al. 1993; P.D. Mueller and Korey 1998; Nimmo et al. 1993; L. Roberts and Wright 1993; Screaton et al. 1992; Singarajah and Lavies 1992; Smilkstein et al. 1987). Five of these cases were fatal. The effect of MDMA on serotonin neurotransmission is discussed later in the section "Pathogenesis." The onset of the serotonin syndrome in most cases described above was with within several hours to several days of administration of serotoninergic medications or dosage increase.

Clinical Variables

Other than the risks associated with MAOI-tricyclic and MAOI-SRI combinations, there are no other known risk factors for the development of the serotonin syndrome (Keck and Arnold 2000). In addition to pharmacodynamic interactions, pharmacokinetic interactions appear to have contributed to the development of the syndrome in several cases. Specifically, these reports suggest that the administration of serotoninergic agents with other medications (with or without direct effects on serotoninergic activity) that substantially inhibit their metabolism may have produced robust increases in the plasma concentrations (Bhatara et al. 1998; Chan et al. 1998; Dingemanse et al. 1998).

Most cases of the syndrome have occurred in patients with psychiatric disorders for which serotoninergic agents are commonly prescribed (e.g., mood disorders, obsessive-compulsive disorder, panic disorder, and generalized anxiety disorder). The syndrome also has been reported in patients with migraine (Blier and Bergeron 1995; Joffe and Sokolov 1997; Mathew et al. 1996), Parkinson's disease (Richard et al. 1997; Sandyk 1986; Weiss 1995), and MDMA intoxication (P.D. Mueller and Korey 1998) and in unintentional overdoses in children (Bedford Russell et al. 1992; Horowitz and Mullins 1999; Pao and Tipnis 1997). Of the cases reported in the scientific literature since 1991, the mean (SD) age was 43 (12) (range = 13 months–82 years); 53 (31.5%) of 168 cases were in men. This disproportionate sex ratio is likely to be due to the higher prevalence of mood disorder and migraine in women. In contrast to NMS, no evidence to date suggests that the physiological state of the patient may contribute to the development of the serotonin syndrome.

🌀 Clinical and Laboratory Features

Clinical Features

The clinical features of the serotonin syndrome include alterations in mental status and behavior, hyperthermia, and signs and symptoms of neurological, gastrointestinal, and autonomic nervous system dysfunction (Table 3–2). In general, substantial heterogeneity in the signs and symptoms of the serotonin syndrome is found across cases reported. This heterogeneity is likely a result of the degree of detail provided in cases reported and differences in severity among cases. Altered mental status was reported in all but 25 (14.9%) of the 168 cases reported in the literature since 1991. Mental status changes included alterations in level of consciousness (e.g., confusion, delirium, and coma) and mood (e.g., hypomania, irritability, anxiety, and dysphoria). Behavioral abnormalities were also common, with restlessness described in 55 (32.7%) cases and agitation in 43 (25.6%) others. The emergence and severity of autonomic nervous system disturbances appeared to parallel the severity of the syndrome. These signs and symptoms included tachycardia, labile blood pressure changes, diaphoresis, shivering, tachypnea, mydriasis, and sialorrhea. Hyperthermia also was associated with severity of the syndrome and was reported in 53 (31.5%) cases. The high proportion of patients with hyperthermia may reflect a reporting bias toward more severe cases. Neurological signs of serotonin syndrome were tremor, myoclonus, ankle clonus, muscle rigidity, hyperreflexia, ataxia, and incoordination. Interestingly, gastrointestinal signs and symptoms were not commonly observed.

Laboratory Findings

No specific laboratory abnormalities have been identified in association with the serotonin syndrome. Those that have been reported have been

TABLE 3–2.   Clinical features of the serotonin syndrome

Mental status
  Anxiety
  Confusion
  Delirium
  Dysphoria
  Hypomania
  Irritability

Behavioral
  Agitation
  Restlessness

Autonomic nervous system
  Diaphoresis
  Hypertension
  Hypotension
  Mydriasis
  Shivering
  Sialorrhea
  Tachycardia
  Tachypnea

Neurological
  Ankle clonus
  Ataxia and incoordination
  Hyperreflexia
  Muscle rigidity
  Myoclonus
  Tremor

Gastrointestinal
  Diarrhea
  Incontinence
  Nausea
  Vomiting

Hyperthermia

Source.   Adapted from Keck PE Jr, Arnold LM: "Serotonin Syndrome." *Psychiatric Annals* 30:333–343, 2000. Used with permission.

either nonspecific (e.g., leukocytosis) or secondary to complications of the syndrome (e.g., azotemia, thrombocytopenia). However, a thorough laboratory evaluation is often needed to rule out other causes of the clinical features associated with serotonin syndrome, especially in moderate to severe cases (Keck and Arnold 2000; Sternbach 1991). Among the 168 cases described since 1991, leukocytosis was reported in 14 (8.3%) cases. Rhabdomyolysis with associated elevations in creatine phosphokinase (CPK) levels was reported in 45 (26.8%) cases; 7 (4.2%) led to myoglobinuria-induced acute renal failure and death. Elevations of CPK were modest in most cases but were increased 1,000-fold in 12 (7.1%) cases. Findings indicative of disseminated intravascular coagulation (DIC) were reported in 10 (6.0%) cases; 6 were fatal. Similarly, clinically significant hepatic transaminase elevations were reported in only 7 (4.2%) cases, but 5 were fatal. Hyponatremia, hypomagnesemia, and hypercalcemia also have been reported in isolated cases. These abnormalities are likely to be secondary to fluid and electrolyte disturbances resulting from the syndrome.

Environmental Factors

Few data suggest that elevated ambient temperature or other environmental factors posed significant risks in the development of serotonin syndrome among reported cases (Butzkueven 1997). However, J.A. Henry et al. (1992) speculated that MDMA-induced serotonin syndrome may be linked to vigorous physical activity, elevated ambient temperature, and inadequate fluid intake occurring during "rave" parties.

🗿 Diagnosis

Three criteria sets have been proposed to date to define the serotonin syndrome. No formal consensus has yet been achieved regarding the criteria for the syndrome. Sternbach (1991) proposed the first operational criteria based on his review of 38 cases (Table 3–3). Dursun et al. (1993) dropped "tremor" and "diaphoresis" from Sternbach's list of core features but added "restless feet while sitting" (akathisia) and "oculogyric crisis." This group further proposed changing "myoclonus" to "initial involuntary contraction followed by myoclonic-like movements in legs" and "mental status changes" to "frightened, diaphoretic hyperarousal state." These criteria were compared in one study conducted to assess the incidence of serotonin syndrome in patients treated with clomipramine (Kudo et al. 1997). With Sternbach's criteria, 8 (12.1%) of 66 patients met criteria for the syndrome, but only 2 (3.0%) met criteria based on the definition of Dursun et al. (1993). The authors of this comparison study suggested that Sternbach's criteria were more sensitive but possibly less specific, whereas Dursun et al.'s might be less sensitive to milder cases but more specific.

Hegerl et al. (1998) proposed a third definition of serotonin syndrome based on further modifications of Sternbach's criteria. They deleted "shivering" because of its overlap with other items reflective of temperature dysregulation and because of its subjectivity. They also modified "mental status changes" to "disorders of orientation" and added "dizziness." The investigators subsequently developed the nine-item SSS based on their criteria and attempted to study the validity of these criteria in a group of

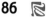

TABLE 3–3. Operational criteria for serotonin syndrome

1. Coincident with the addition of or increase in a known serotoninergic agent to an established medication regimen, at least three of the following clinical features are present:
   - Mental status changes (e.g., confusion or hypomania)
   - Agitation
   - Myoclonus
   - Hyperreflexia
   - Diaphoresis
   - Shivering
   - Tremor
   - Diarrhea
   - Incoordination
   - Fever
2. Other etiologies have been ruled out.
3. A neuroleptic had not been started or increased in dosage prior to the onset of the signs and symptoms listed above.

Source. Adapted from Sternbach H: "The Serotonin Syndrome." *American Journal of Psychiatry* 148:705–713, 1991. Used with permission. Copyright 1991 American Psychiatric Association.

patients receiving paroxetine alone or in combination with other psychotropic agents. As an independent validating measure of serotoninergic activity, they measured serum paroxetine concentrations and the loudness dependence of auditory evoked potentials (LDAEP). The LDAEP response is believed to be inversely correlated with CNS serotoninergic activity. As anticipated, the SSS score positively correlated with serum paroxetine concentrations and negatively with the LDAEP response. When a threshold SSS score of >6 was used, 5 (11.9%) of 42 patients met criteria for mild serotonin syndrome. Interestingly, SSS scores and total Hamilton Rating Scale for Depression scores also positively correlated. This correlation may have been the result of some overlap between symptoms of serotonin syndrome and major depressive disorder (e.g., agitation, dizziness, diarrhea) (Keck and Arnold 2000).

The signs and symptoms of serotonin syndrome reported in the 168 cases since 1991 are comparable with those proposed by Sternbach (1991). This is not surprising because most reports used these criteria to define the syndrome. Nevertheless, of the 10 core features of the syndrome identified by Sternbach, only diarrhea occurred with a low prevalence rate (8%). Other features were reported commonly, including autonomic nervous system dysfunction (e.g., tachycardia, 37%; labile blood pressure changes, 24%; mydriasis, 25%) and muscle rigidity (33%). These data suggest that muscle rigidity and signs of autonomic nervous system instability should be included as criteria for serotonin syndrome and diarrhea omitted. In short, these modified criteria would include

1. Mental status changes
2. Agitation or restlessness
3. Myoclonus
4. Hyperreflexia
5. Diaphoresis
6. Tremor
7. Shivering
8. Incoordination
9. Autonomic nervous system dysfunction
10. Hyperthermia
11. Muscle rigidity

The phenomenological overlap of serotonin syndrome with NMS is apparent in the last three criteria.

🌀 Differential Diagnosis

The diagnosis of serotonin syndrome involves differentiating this condition from other disorders associated with cognitive and behavioral, neuromuscular, and autonomic nervous system dysfunction with or without hyperthermia. Thus, the differential diagnosis of serotonin syndrome is virtually identical to that of and includes NMS (Table 3–4) (Dursun et al. 1995; Miyaoka and Kamijima 1995). In patients receiving antipsychotic and serotoninergic medications, differentiation between the two syndromes can be very difficult (Cassidy and O'Keane 2000; Nimmagadda et al. 2000). The primary clinical features that differentiate serotonin syndrome from NMS are myoclonus, hyperreflexia, shivering, and gastrointestinal symptoms in serotonin syndrome and more frequent and severe manifestations of muscle rigidity in NMS (Keck and Arnold 2000). In addition, hyperthermia, autonomic nervous system dysfunction, leukocytosis, and other laboratory abnormalities appear to occur less consistently and primarily in severe cases of serotonin syndrome. Serotonin syndrome also has characteristics that overlap with carcinoid syndrome, although the latter is more commonly associated with flushing and dyspnea (Trivedi 1984). There is one report of sertraline unmasking carcinoid syndrome (Noyer and Schwartz 1997). Finally, some features of serotonin syndrome occur in the SRI discontinuation syndrome (Rosenbaum et al. 1998). These include mood and mental status changes, diaphoresis, incoordination, diarrhea, and shivering. The SRI discontinuation syndrome

TABLE 3–4.   Features of serotonin syndrome and neuroleptic malignant syndrome

Feature	Serotonin syndrome	Neuroleptic malignant syndrome
Temperature	Hyperthermia variable	Hyperthermia
Mental status	Delirium	Delirium
	Stupor	Stupor
	Confusion	Confusion
	Coma	Coma
	Anxiety	
	Euphoria	
	Irritability	
Neurological	Muscle rigidity variable	Muscle rigidity
	Hyperreflexia	Hyperreflexia uncommon
	Tremor	Tremor
	Ankle clonus	
	Myoclonus	
	Incoordination	
Behavioral	Agitation	Agitation
	Restlessness	Restlessness
Autonomic	Diaphoresis	Diaphoresis
	Tachycardia	Tachycardia
	Tachypnea	Tachypnea
	Hyper- or hypotension	Hyper- or hypotension
	Incontinence	Incontinence
	Mydriasis	Mydriasis
	Sialorrhea	Sialorrhea
	Shivering	
Gastrointestinal	Diarrhea	
	Nausea	
	Vomiting	
Laboratory	Elevations uncommon:	Elevations common:
	Creatine phosphokinase	Creatine phosphokinase
	White blood cell count	White blood cell count
	Liver function tests	Liver function tests

Source.   Adapted from Keck PE Jr, Arnold LM: "Serotonin Syndrome." *Psychiatric Annals* 30:333–343, 2000. Used with permission.

typically follows abrupt cessation of SRI medications and has not been reported to be associated with hyperthermia, significant autonomic nervous system dysfunction, myoclonus, or muscle rigidity.

Complications

In most reports, serotonin syndrome has been mild to moderate in severity without medical complications. However, a distinct minority of cases, particularly those associated with MAOI-tricyclic and MAOI-SRI combinations and MDMA, were severe and some fatal. Overall, medical complications appear to be less common than in NMS. Rhabdomyolysis was the most common serious medical complication of serotonin syndrome, occurring in 45 (26.8%) cases. Myoglobinuria and renal failure were reported in 8 (4.8%) patients. Generalized seizures were reported in 18 (10.7%) cases, including 7 fatalities. Similarly, DIC occurred in 8 patients, 5 of whom died. Thus, although medical complications were not common in patients with serotonin syndrome, they were associated with a substantial mortality risk.

🍵 Pathogenesis

Excessive serotoninergic neurotransmission appears to be the basis of serotonin syndrome. Preclinical studies performed decades ago were the first to identify the role of serotonin in this syndrome. A toxic serotonin syndrome in animals occurred when serotoninergic stimulation was enhanced by direct stimulation of serotonin receptors with serotonin agonists or administration of combinations of L-tryptophan or SRIs with MAOIs (Gerson and Baldessarini 1980). The features of this syndrome presaged human manifestations of serotonin syndrome and included tremor, rigidity, hypertonicity, hyperreactivity, myoclonus, generalized seizures, and autonomic nervous system dysfunction. The next step in elucidating the pathophysiology of the syndrome was to identify the relevant serotonin receptors involved in the interaction. In preclinical studies, the postsynaptic serotonin type 1A (5-HT_{1A}) receptor appeared to mediate many features of the serotonin syndrome (L.M. Smith and Peroutka 1986) (see Chapter 2), although the head-twitch response seems related to overstimulation of 5-HT_{2A} receptors. Notably, as detailed in Chapter 2, hyperthermia in serotonin syndrome also appears mediated by 5-HT_{2A} receptors (Nisijima et al. 2001). Furthermore, stimulation of the 5-HT_3 receptor may be involved in causing the syndrome's gastrointestinal manifestations (Kishibayashi et al. 1993).

    In humans, the greatest concentration of serotoninergic neuron cell bodies is found in the brain stem nuclei, primarily the dorsal and median raphe, which project to the septum, hippocampus, entorhinal cortex, cerebral cortex, thalamic and hypothalamic nuclei, and interpeduncular nucleus (Ivanusa et al. 1997). Projections to hypothalamic nuclei may mediate hyperthermic reactions in severe cases of the serotonin syndrome. Serotoninergic neurons are also involved in the enervation of respiratory muscles and regulation of cardiac functions. In animals, the peripheral manifestations of the serotonin syndrome appear to be mediated primarily by 5-HT$_{1A}$ receptors in the lower brain stem and spinal cord (Jacobs and Klemfuss 1975). Lauterbach (1998) suggested that excess serotoninergic stimulation of 5-HT$_{1A}$ receptors may be involved in the development of catatonia. Carroll (2000) proposed that this mechanism also may be involved in the pathophysiology of NMS. Ascending serotoninergic projections almost certainly play a role, particularly in the mood and mental status changes and thermoregulatory dysregulation of the syndrome. Catecholamines and other serotonin receptors also may contribute to the syndrome, but their roles are unclear (Renyi 1991).

The role of MDMA in precipitating the serotonin syndrome in a few fatal cases deserves special scrutiny. MDMA produces a massive release of serotonin, depleting presynaptic stores by as much as 80% within 4 hours after a single injection (Gillman 1997a). MDMA also may produce enduring neurotoxic effects (Ricaurte et al. 1988). Semple et al. (1999) found a cortical reduction in serotonin transporter binding by using single photon emission computed tomography (SPECT) in regular Ecstasy users compared with healthy control subjects. This reduction in serotonin transporter binding was especially prominent in primary sensorimotor cortex and provided additional evidence for specific serotoninergic neurotoxicity of MDMA. Gerra et al. (2000) also found evidence of enduring impairment in central serotoninergic functioning in a study of prolactin and cortisol responses to D-fenfluramine in MDMA abusers. These data suggest that serotonin syndrome precipitated by MDMA may be especially severe because of massive surges in serotonin release in an otherwise hypofunctioning serotoninergic system.

Treatment

No systematic studies of the treatment of serotonin syndrome have been done. In most of the cases reported, the syndrome was self-limited and usually resolved quickly after discontinuation of serotoninergic medications. In more severe cases, other interventions were necessary. These included respiratory and cardiovascular monitoring and support, the use of a cooling blanket for hyperthermia, intravenous hydration to prevent renal failure, and anticonvulsants for myoclonus or seizures. Drug discontinuation and supportive measures were associated with resolution of the syndrome in 74 (44.0%) of the 168 cases reported since those reviewed by Sternbach (1991). In most of these cases, patients had mild to moderate signs and symptoms of the syndrome.

The use of specific pharmacological treatments is anecdotal but can be considered in severe cases of serotonin syndrome or in patients who do not respond to discontinuation of serotoninergic agents and supportive measures (Keck and Arnold 2000; Lane and Baldwin 1997; Sporer 1995; Sternbach 1991). The nonspecific serotonin antagonist cyproheptadine (4–24 mg/day) was the most consistently effective treatment in case reports, with rapid resolution occurring in 19 (90.5%) of 21 patients (Chan et al. 1998; Diamond et al. 1998; George and Godleski 1996; Goldberg and Huk 1992; Graudins et al. 1998; Lappin and Auchincloss 1994; Muly et al. 1993; Roxanas and Machado 1998). Benzodiazepines were administered in 33 cases (Bastani et al. 1996; Brannan et al. 1994; Brodribb et al. 1995; Brubacher et al. 1996; Butzkueven 1997; Chan et al. 1998; Graudins et al. 1998; Heisler et al. 1996; Hodgman et al. 1997; Hoes and Zeijpveld 1996; John et al. 1997; Klaassen et al. 1998; Lappin and Auchincloss 1994; Lejoyeux et al. 1992; Mekler and Woggon 1997; Nierenberg and Semprebon 1993; Rella and Hoffman 1998; Skop et al. 1994; Spigset and Adielsson 1997; A.L. Weiner et al. 1997; L.A. Weiner et al. 1998) and appeared to be effective in 5, of equivocal benefit in 19, and of no benefit in 9. Low-potency typical antipsychotics were tried in 6 cases, all with equivocal benefit (Chan et al. 1998; Daniels 1998; Diamond et al. 1998; Gillman 1996; Grantham et al. 1964). However, the use of neuroleptics in a patient with suspected serotonin syndrome could complicate the subsequent course of illness and pose a theoretical risk of exacerbating hyperthermia.

Several other agents, including propranolol (L-isomer is a serotonin antagonist) (Guze and Baxter 1986; Heisler et al. 1996; Lappin and Auchincloss 1994), ketanserin (a 5-HT_2 antagonist) (Klassen et al. 1998), and mirtazapine (5-HT_2 and 5-HT_3 antagonist) (Hoes and Zeijpveld 1996) produced equivocal improvement in a few cases. Mirtazapine also was suspected of contributing to the development of serotonin syndrome (Benazzi 1997). Nitroglycerin was reported effective in one case (T.M. Brown and Skop 1996). Dantrolene, a muscle relaxant thought to be effective in treating NMS (Nisijima and Ishiguro 1995b), was administered in 10 patients (9 severe); 4 (40%) of the 10 patients appeared to improve markedly (Butzkueven 1997; Demirkiran et al. 1996; Graber et al. 1994; Hodgman et al. 1997; John et al. 1997; Keltner and Harris 1994; L.A. Weiner et al. 1998). In contrast to the clinical data and based on an animal model of serotonin syndrome, Nisijima et al. (2001) argued that potent 5-HT_{2A} receptor antagonists (including atypical antipsychotics) represent the most effective drugs for treating this condition. This view derives from the role of 5-HT_{2A} receptors in mediating hyperthermia and the association of hyperthermia with severity of the syndrome.

🗐 Conclusion

The serotonin syndrome is an uncommon adverse event usually produced by combinations or high doses of serotoninergic medications. The features of the syndrome include mental status and mood changes, behavioral and neuromuscular abnormalities, autonomic nervous system dysfunction, and hyperthermia. The onset of the syndrome is usually abrupt following the addition of or increase in the dose of a serotoninergic agent. In many cases, the syndrome is mild and abates when serotoninergic agents are discontinued. The most severe cases have been associated with MAOI-tricyclic and MAOI-SRI combinations and MDMA abuse. In severe cases, rapid intervention with supportive measures may be required, and nonspecific serotonin antagonists may be helpful. The development of a 5-HT_{1A} antagonist could provide a more specific pharmacological intervention, and the utility of 5-HT_{2A} antagonists merits further investigation. Despite heightened clinical awareness in recent years, recent surveys suggest that the syndrome still may be underdiagnosed. Greater awareness of the drug combinations commonly associated with the syndrome should lead to better prevention and early recognition and treatment.

CHAPTER 4

Hyperthermia Associated With Other Neuropsychiatric Drugs

As discussed in the preceding chapters, data obtained from clinical and animal studies convincingly implicate neuroleptic drugs in disorders of thermoregulation, including neuroleptic malignant syndrome (NMS) and heatstroke. In addition to neuroleptics, other neuropsychiatric drugs have been implicated in the development of hyperthermic syndromes. In this chapter, an overview of the clinical aspects and theoretical mechanisms of these rare hyperthermic syndromes is presented. The occurrence of hyperthermia in relation to antidepressants has generated a large body of literature, which is covered in Chapter 3 on the serotonin syndrome. Clarification of the clinical manifestations of these drug-related conditions is essential in determining their resemblance to NMS. Recognition of similar features would be clinically relevant in terms of differential diagnosis and, conceivably, may broaden investigations of common pathophysiological mechanisms.

☜ Hypodopaminergic Syndromes

In recent years, an increasing number of clinical reports have come to light in which NMS-like conditions were described in patients taking agents other than neuroleptics, which could directly affect activity in dopaminergic systems in the brain. Since these cases are unrelated to neuroleptic use per se, they are not, by definition, examples of NMS. However, these cases provide compelling evidence supporting the hypothesis that an acute reduction in central dopamine activity may be a primary etiological mechanism in the development of NMS.

V.W. Henderson and Wooten (1981) first reported this phenomenon in a 50-year-old patient with Parkinson's disease who developed NMS symptoms 2 days after treatment with carbidopa/levodopa, amantadine, and diphenhydramine was discontinued. Subsequent reports have confirmed that a syndrome consisting of mental status changes, severe extrapyramidal symptoms, autonomic disturbances, and hyperthermia may occur following withdrawal of dopamine agonists in patients with Parkinson's disease (Cunningham et al. 1991; Figa-Talamanca et al. 1985; J.H. Friedman et al. 1985; Gibb 1988; Gordon and Frucht 2001; Iwasaki et al. 1992; Keyser and Rodnitzky 1991; Lazarus et al. 1989; Rainer et al. 1991; Rascol et al. 1990; Sechi et al. 1984; Ueda et al. 1999, 2001). Rhabdomyolysis with serum levels of creatine phosphokinase (CPK) as high as 50,000 IU also has been reported as part of this syndrome (J.H. Friedman et al. 1985). Furthermore, like NMS, it may be life threatening; three deaths have been reported (Gibb 1988; Sechi et al. 1984).

Most often, this reaction has been observed when carbidopa/levodopa was withdrawn from patients with Parkinson's disease because of lack of response, severe dyskinesias, or psychosis. In these cases, the duration of antiparkinsonian treatment ranged from 6 months to 10 years. The onset of the syndrome followed termination of drug therapy in 1–7 days. In some cases, anticholinergic drugs were discontinued along with levodopa, and this may have potentiated an imbalance of neurotransmitters in the extrapyramidal system. However, in other cases, continuation of anticholinergics had little discernible effect on the evolution of the reaction (Burke et al. 1981). Apart from levodopa, withdrawal of other dopamine-enhancing drugs also has resulted in NMS-like symptoms in patients receiving treatment for Parkinson's disease (Bower et al. 1994; Iwuagwu and Bonomo 2000; D.M. Simpson and Davis 1984).

In several additional cases, NMS-like symptoms developed in patients with Parkinson's disease even though dopaminergic therapy was continued without changes in dosage (Cao and Katz 1999; J.H. Friedman et al. 1985; Kuno et al. 1997; Pfeiffer and Sucha 1985; Y. Yamawaki and Ogawa 1992). In cases reported by J.H. Friedman et al. (1985) and Pfeiffer and Sucha (1985), a fatal NMS-like condition developed during "off" episodes in patients with Parkinson's disease while treatment with carbidopa/levodopa was maintained. Although the exact mechanism underlying the "on-off" phenomenon is unknown, available evidence suggests that off periods correlate with troughs of plasma concentrations and striatal activity of levodopa (Quinn 1987). In the case reported by Pfeiffer and Sucha (1985), the reaction occurred in a patient who was also taking lithium (900 mg) daily, which had been prescribed in an attempt to ameliorate episodes of "freezing" associated with maintenance levodopa therapy (Reches and Fahn 1983). Noting the resemblance of the reaction in this patient to reports of hyperthermia related to lithium-neuroleptic combinations, Pfeiffer and Sucha (1985) suggested that lithium should be used cautiously in Parkinson's disease patients experiencing "on-off" fluctuations.

In addition to intensive, supportive care, treatment to date usually has consisted of reintroduction of dopamine agonists and anticholinergic drugs, although this pharmacological strategy did not prevent a fatal outcome in four patients (Gibb 1988; Rainer et al. 1991; Sechi et al. 1984). In one case, dantrolene was used successfully in combination with levodopa and bromocriptine in the management of NMS-like symptoms (Figa-Talamanca et al. 1985).

Similar NMS-like reactions, related to either pharmacological or idiopathic reduction of dopamine activity, have been reported in patients with Huntington's disease, influenza A encephalopathy, acute hydrocephalus, striatonigral degeneration, Hallervorden-Spatz disease, multisystem atrophy, Shy-Drager syndrome, Lewy body dementia, and progressive supranuclear palsy (Hayashi et al. 1993; Ito et al. 2001; M. Itoh et al. 1995; Komatsu et al. 1992; Konagaya et al. 1997; Kumagai et al. 1998; Lazarus et al. 1989; Lu and Ryu 1991; Sechi et al. 2000; Yoshikawa et al. 1997). In these disorders, treatment usually has included dopaminergic agonists, which were combined with dantrolene in a few cases.

As discussed in Chapter 1, several drugs prescribed in clinical practice have central antidopaminergic properties but are not administered for antipsychotic effect (Caroff and Mann 1993; Caroff et al. 2001a, 2001c). Nevertheless, NMS has been reported in association with such drugs, including droperidol, promethazine, prochlorperazine, reserpine, and metoclopramide (Caroff et al. 2001c).

Among antidepressants, amoxapine, an *N*-desmethyl analogue of loxapine, a dibenzoxepine antipsychotic, also has been associated with hyperthermia, rigidity, and rhabdomyolysis during treatment with therapeutic doses (Burch and Downs 1987; Lesaca 1987; Steele 1982) as well as when taken in overdose (Litovitz and Troutman 1983; N.E. Taylor and Schwartz 1988). Some of these cases have been considered examples of NMS (Coccaro and Siever 1985). However, unlike NMS, prolonged seizures that occurred following amoxapine overdose may have contributed to heat generation (Wachtel et al. 1987). Furthermore, the relation between hyperthermia, rigidity, rhabdomyolysis, seizures, and acute renal failure in these cases is inconsistent so that common mechanisms underlying these manifestations are unclear (Abreo et al. 1982; Jennings et al. 1983; Pumariega et al. 1982). Yet the resemblance of cases of amoxapine toxicity to NMS is not surprising because amoxapine and its 7-hydroxy metabolite possess potent dopamine receptor antagonist properties in addition to effects on noradrenergic, serotoninergic, and cholinergic systems (Coccaro and Siever 1985; Steele 1982).

Pathogenesis

These cases show that, in addition to NMS, which is associated with neuroleptic-induced dopamine receptor blockade, potentially life-threatening hyperthermic reactions may occur following administration of dopamine-depleting drugs, following withdrawal of dopamine agonists, or as a result of functional changes in dopamine activity during off episodes in Parkinson's disease. Thus, inhibition of dopamine transmission, regardless of etiology, appears to be a common mechanism underlying these reactions.

Furthermore, because the neurodegenerative process in Parkinson's disease and systematically administered dopamine agonists and antagonists presumably affect the cortex, limbic system, and hypothalamus in addition to the basal ganglia, concurrent dysfunction in several dopamine pathways may be necessary for the development of NMS-like symptoms. In fact, inhibition of dopamine activity in mesocortical and mesolimbic tracts has been invoked to explain cognitive decline, autonomic dysfunction, and impairment of thermoregulation in Parkinson's disease (Lazarus et al. 1989). Although changes in other neurotransmitter systems—including norepinephrine, serotonin, acetylcholine, γ-aminobutyric acid (GABA), and neuropeptides—have been reported in Parkinson's disease (Voigt and Uhl 1987; Wooten 1987), their clinical significance in relation to motor symptoms and hyperthermia remains unclear.

The importance of central dopaminergic hypoactivity in NMS-like episodes reported in Parkinson's disease is also supported by the work of Ueda and colleagues (1999, 2001). These investigators found that patients with Parkinson's disease who developed NMS-like symptoms during or following withdrawal from dopaminergic therapy showed significantly lower levels of homovanillic acid (HVA) in the cerobrospinal fluid during and after the episode compared with control subjects. They also observed that patients who developed NMS-like symptoms were more likely to be dehydrated, to have more severe parkinsonian disability, and to experience "wearing off" fluctuations. Consistent with reports related to NMS (Rosebush and Mazurek 1991), Iwasaki et al. (1992) reported reduced plasma iron during an NMS-like syndrome that followed dopamine agonist withdrawal in a patient with Parkinson's disease. Finally, Kuno et al. (1997) suggested that high ambient temperatures, dehydration, and premenstrual worsening of parkinsonian symptoms contributed to the onset of the syndrome in a case series of 19 patients.

The development of animal models, which could be used to investigate dopamine-mediated hyperthermic syndromes, may be facilitated by investigations of the parkinsonian state in substance abusers inadvertently exposed to 1-methyl-4-phenyl-1,2,3,6-tetrahydropyridine (MPTP) (Ballard et al. 1985; Burns et al. 1983, 1985; Heikkila et al. 1987; Jenner and Marsden 1986; Kopin 1987). Although elevated serum CPK and diaphoresis have been occasionally reported (Ballard et al. 1985), hyperthermia has not been observed in humans or animals exposed to this neurotoxin. This is puzzling because the rapid onset of parkinsonism associated with destruction of dopamine-containing neurons by MPTP would seem to parallel the acute development of hyperthermia in susceptible patients treated with neuroleptics or withdrawn from dopamine agonists. However, MPTP-induced parkinsonism is unique; MPTP selectively damages dopamine neurons in the zona compacta of the substantia nigra, whereas the neuropathology of idiopathic Parkinson's disease is multifocal, and the effects of dopamine agonists and antagonists are similarly not limited to the nigrostriatal tract (Heikkila et al. 1987; Jenner and Marsden 1986). In addition, degenerative changes in other neurotransmitter systems reported in the idiopathic disease may not occur in MPTP-induced parkinsonism (Ballard et al. 1985; Burns et al. 1985; Heikkila et al. 1987; Jenner and Marsden 1986). However, transient functional changes in extrastriatal dopamine, and norepinephrine and serotonin, associated with acute behavioral effects reminiscent of the "serotonin syndrome" (Jacobs 1976; Jacobs and Kleinfuss 1975) have been reported after MPTP administration (Burns et al. 1983; Kopin 1987).

🔏 Baclofen

There are several very interesting reports of NMS-like features emerging in patients withdrawn from baclofen, a GABA agonist (Khorasani and Peruzzi 1995; Mandac et al. 1993; R.K. Reeves et al. 1998; Samson-Fang et al. 2000; Siegfried et al. 1992; M.R. Turner and Gainsborough 2001). Episodes consisting of hyperthermia, hypertonicity of skeletal muscles, mental status changes, autonomic changes, respiratory distress, rhabdomyolysis, and disseminated intravascular coagulation (DIC) have been reported in patients withdrawn from oral (Mandac et al. 1993; M.R. Turner and Gainsborough 2001) and intrathecal baclofen (Khorasani and Peruzzi

1995; R.K. Reeves et al. 1998; Samson-Fang et al. 2000; Siegfried et al. 1992). Besides supportive care, treatment has included reinstitution of baclofen treatment and even dantrolene in two cases (Khorasani and Peruzzi 1995; R.K. Reeves et al. 1998).

Implications of these reports for understanding the pathogenesis of hyperthermic conditions are potentially significant. These cases of baclofen withdrawal leading to GABA deficiency are consistent with reports of reduced GABA levels in the cerebrospinal fluid of NMS patients (Nisijima and Ishiguro 1995a), the efficacy of GABA-ergic drugs and electroconvulsive therapy in treating NMS (J.M. Davis et al. 2000), and GABA-dopamine interactions in the pathogenesis of these syndromes (Fricchione et al. 2000).

Another puzzling aspect of these cases is the development of a systemic hypermetabolic state despite previous spinal cord transections. In the absence of upper motor neuron input, these patients developed NMS-like syndromes, suggesting that spinal or peripheral mechanisms may play a role in the production of hypermetabolism and hyperthermia.

🗿 Lithium

Neurotoxicity related to treatment with lithium has been recognized for many years. A broad range of effects on both central and peripheral components of the nervous system has been described. In states of mild intoxication, vomiting and diarrhea may be accompanied by apathy, lethargy, weakness, and a worsening tremor. With severe intoxication, an acute encephalopathy may develop, characterized by mental confusion, ataxia, dysarthria, gross tremor, choreoathetoid movements, myoclonus, parkinsonism, hyperreflexia, cranial nerve and other focal signs, seizures, coma, and death. Encephalopathy due to lithium toxicity is often accompanied by slowing of the dominant rhythm on electroencephalogram (EEG) (Sansone and Ziegler 1985).

Some investigators have found that neurotoxicity may occur at serum levels of lithium in the therapeutic range, perhaps because of variation in sensitivity or relatively greater concentrations of lithium in brain tissue in some patients (Evans and Garner 1979; Jefferson et al. 1987; Sansone and Ziegler 1985). In addition, it has been suggested that elderly patients, patients with underlying brain disease, and patients treated with other psychotropic drugs may be at risk for developing lithium neurotoxicity.

The mortality rate following serious lithium overdose approaches 15% (Hansen and Amdisen 1978; Schou 1984; Tesio et al. 1987), but an additional 10% of patients appear to be at risk for irreversible neurological damage (Prakash et al. 1982; Sansone and Ziegler 1985; Tesio et al. 1987).

Most often, patients are left with cerebellar abnormalities and movement disorders, although changes in cortical functions (e.g., diminished short-term memory) (Apte and Langston 1983; Schou 1984) and evidence of peripheral neuropathy (Schou 1984) have been described. In a review of cases with neurological sequelae, Schou (1984) found that some improvement could be expected 6–12 months after intoxication, whereas change was unlikely to occur after 1 year.

Hyperthermia, as reported in NMS, is not typical of lithium neurotoxicity, although lithium was associated with heatstroke in one case (Lowance 1980), and fever has been reported in comatose patients usually in association with intercurrent infection (Tesio et al. 1987). However, in four patients, fever was associated with lithium treatment in the absence of signs of infection or intoxication (Ananth and Ruskin 1974; G.P. Downey et al. 1984; Gabuzda and Frankenburg 1987). Susman and Addonizio (1987) reported recurrence of NMS symptomatology in two patients treated with therapeutic doses of lithium just after recovery from NMS; the investigators noted that the proximity of neuroleptic exposure in these cases suggests that toxicity may have resulted from the lithium-neuroleptic combination rather than the effects of lithium alone.

In addition to reports of encephalopathy, and rare instances of hyperthermia, some investigators have focused specifically on extrapyramidal effects of lithium (Asnis et al. 1979; Branchey et al. 1976; Johnels et al. 1976; Sansone and Ziegler 1985; Shopsin and Gershon 1975; Tyrer et al. 1980). In all of these reports, the extrapyramidal changes were mild, and the causal relation with lithium may have been complicated by prior exposure to neuroleptics (Jefferson et al. 1987). Nevertheless, these cases suggest that lithium may have clinically significant effects on the extrapyramidal system.

Conflicting data concerning extrapyramidal effects of lithium have emerged from clinical reports describing the use of lithium in the treatment of tardive dyskinesia. Although lithium has been reported to delay the development and reduce the severity of tardive dyskinesia (Gerlach et al. 1975; Reda et al. 1975), others have found that lithium exerts no significant effect on tardive dyskinesia (Foti and Pies 1986; Jus et al. 1978; G.M. Simpson et al. 1976; Yassa et al. 1984) or may even exacerbate the movement disorder (Beitman 1978; Crews and Carpenter 1977; Himmelhoch et al. 1980; Jefferson et al. 1987).

Similarly, there have been conflicting reports on the efficacy of lithium in the prophylactic management of "freezing" episodes in patients with Parkinson's disease maintained on levodopa (Coffey et al. 1982; Jefferson et al. 1987; Lieberman and Gopinathan 1982; Pfeiffer and Sucha 1985; Reches and Fahn 1983).

Finally, lithium affects the peripheral nervous system at therapeutic and toxic doses. As with central effects, peripheral toxicity may be enhanced in patients with preexisting neuromuscular disorders (Sansone and Ziegler 1985). Flaccid paralysis, proximal muscle weakness, fasciculations, and areflexia usually accompany lithium-induced encephalopathy. There have been isolated reports of myopathy (Julien et al. 1979) and myasthenia gravis–like illnesses (Dilsaver 1987; Neil et al. 1976) in lithium-treated patients. Rhabdomyolysis is unusual but was reported in a single case with many of the features of NMS (Unger et al. 1982). However, the role of concurrently administered drugs in this case was not entirely clear. Lithium appears to potentiate neuromuscular blockade by pancuronium and succinylcholine during anesthesia (Jefferson et al. 1987), perhaps by reducing acetylcholine synthesis at the nerve terminal (Vizi et al. 1972) or by downregulating acetylcholine receptors at the neuromuscular junction (Dilsaver 1987; Pestronk and Drachman 1980). Lithium also has been associated with the development of a reversible neuropathy (Brust et al. 1979; Newman and Saunders 1979) and the reduction of motor nerve conduction velocity (Girke et al. 1975).

Lithium-Neuroleptic Combinations

Lithium is often used in combination with neuroleptics in the treatment of mania. Although this combination has proven valuable and been well tolerated by most patients, there has been continuing controversy over the potential for synergistic neurotoxicity. Some investigators have reported that lithium potentiates extrapyramidal symptoms in patients concurrently receiving neuroleptics (Addonizio 1985; Sachdev 1986).

A more severe form of neurotoxicity in patients receiving lithium and neuroleptics has been described. W.J. Cohen and Cohen (1974) reported a severe encephalopathic syndrome arising in four patients during the course of treatment with haloperidol and lithium. These investigators described this syndrome, which resulted in irreversible brain damage, as consisting of lethargy, fever, tremors, confusion, and extrapyramidal and cerebellar dysfunction accompanied by leukocytosis and elevated serum enzymes, blood urea nitrogen, and glucose. They suggested that these reactions were unlikely to result from either drug alone and proposed that lithium and haloperidol acted synergistically on neuronal metabolic or membrane functions.

In response to this alarming report, some investigators suggested that these cases were artifactual, were due to factors other than drugs, represented inappropriate use of the drugs, or were explainable on the basis of toxicity of either drug alone (Jefferson and Greist 1980; Shopsin et al. 1976; Tupin and Schuller 1978). In addition, several investigators reviewed series of patients treated with combined medications and were unable to find examples of severe neurotoxicity (Abrams and Taylor 1979; Baastrup et al. 1976; Biederman et al. 1979; Goldney and Spence 1986; Growe et al. 1979; Juhl et al. 1977; Krishna et al. 1978; Shopsin et al. 1976; Small et al. 1975).

In contrast, Miller and Menninger (1987b) found evidence of neurotoxicity consisting of delirium, extrapyramidal symptoms, and ataxia in 6 (27.3%) of 22 bipolar patients treated with lithium and neuroleptics. In an expanded retrospective study, these same investigators reported the development of similar neurotoxic changes in 8 (19.5%) of 41 patients receiving concurrent treatment (Miller and Menninger 1987a). Although these findings by Miller and Menninger (1987a, 1987b) were refuted by Kessel et al. (1992), unexpected and severe toxicity, sometimes resulting in persistent neurological damage, has continued to be described in sporadic case reports of patients taking lithium and neuroleptics (Donaldson and Cunningham 1983; Izzo and Brody 1985; Mann et al. 1983; Sandyk and Hurwitz 1983; J. Sellers et al. 1982; C.J. Thomas 1979). In a review of 39 case reports, Prakash et al. (1982) found that 76.3% of such cases occurred in patients treated with neuroleptics and lithium for mood disorders, although in some cases schizophrenia and mental retardation were the principal diagnoses. In cases of toxicity attributed to the lithium-neuroleptic combination, women outnumbered men by a factor of 2 or 3 to 1. The ages ranged from 16 to 64 years, with a mean (±SD) of 46±12 years (Prakash et al. 1982).

Haloperidol was involved in 67% of the cases of combined neurotoxicity, but other neuroleptics that were implicated include fluphenazine, perphenazine, flupenthixol, thiothixene, chlorpromazine, and thioridazine (Prakash et al. 1982). Prakash et al. (1982) reported a wide range (63–32,500 mg) of neuroleptic dosages, expressed in chlorpromazine equivalents, with a median daily dose of 1,346 mg.

In reviewing 21 reported cases of combined neurotoxicity associated with haloperidol, we found that the mean (±SD) daily dose of haloperidol (16.9±12.8 g) was well within the standard therapeutic range. Miller and Menninger (1987a, 1987b) found a correlation between neurotoxicity and the dosage of neuroleptic administered, although the dosages used were believed to be "suitable" therapeutic doses by these investigators. Similarly, in most cases, lithium dosing was within the standard range; in more than 90% of the cases, the serum lithium level at the time of the reaction was below 1.5 mEq/L (Prakash et al. 1982). Thus, these reactions are not explained simply as a function of excessive dosing of either drug.

The manifestations of neurotoxicity in these cases reflect a spectrum of neuropathic features, including stupor, delirium, catatonia, rigidity, ataxia, dysarthria, myoclonus, seizures, and fever. Although W.J. Cohen and Cohen (1974) suggested that this acute encephalopathic picture did not occur with lithium or neuroleptics alone, this is clearly inaccurate, because some of these cases were indistinguishable from NMS. In fact, separation of these cases from NMS is often arbitrary. Many reviewers have included them among series of NMS cases such that 10%–20% of reported cases of NMS have been associated with the administration of lithium in addition to neuroleptics (Caroff and Mann 1988; Kurlan et al. 1984; Levenson 1985; Pearlman 1986). This suggests that some cases of neurotoxicity attributed to combined therapy may actually represent cases of NMS with lithium playing a secondary role. Among reported NMS cases in which lithium was coadministered with neuroleptics, we found no difference in sex, age, symptoms, and outcome compared with NMS cases associated with the use of neuroleptics alone (Caroff and Mann 1988).

However, in their review of 39 patients treated with combined pharmacotherapy and not diagnosed as having NMS, Prakash et al. (1982) found that, unlike NMS cases, a predominance of women were affected. Furthermore, although they reported no deaths, there was a significant risk (11% of cases) of irreversible neurological deficits. Persistent evidence of dementia has been reported in follow-up from 3 to 10 months in at least four patients (W.J. Cohen and Cohen 1974; Sandyk and Hurwitz 1983; C.J. Thomas 1979), and persistent signs of cerebellar or extrapyramidal damage were observed in these four patients and in additional patients followed up for 5–24 months (Donaldson and Cunningham 1983; Izzo and Brody 1985; Mann et al. 1983; J. Sellers et al. 1982; Spring 1979). By comparison, persistent neurological sequelae in NMS survivors are less commonly reported (S.A. Anderson and Weinschenk 1987; Rothke and Bush 1986; Shalev and Munitz 1986; Tenenbein 1986).

Thus, whereas some cases of combined neurotoxicity resemble NMS, other cases are composed of features characteristic of lithium neurotoxicity (Hansen and Amdisen 1978; Sansone and Ziegler 1985; Schou 1984). In fact, several cases of toxicity associated with combined therapy have been attributed to lithium alone (Brust et al. 1979; Donaldson and Cunningham 1983; Izzo and Brody 1985; Rifkin et al. 1973; J. Sellers et al. 1982).

Spring and Frankel (1981) proposed that two types of lithium-neuroleptic toxicity may occur: 1) an NMS-like reaction associated with haloperidol and other high-potency neuroleptics and 2) a primarily lithium-induced reaction associated with phenothiazines, especially thioridazine. This dichotomy is consistent with differences in photic response and EEG findings observed between the groups by Saran et al. (1989). Although several cases fit these two categories, many have features of both, suggesting that adverse reactions to combination therapy may form a continuum of neurotoxicity ranging from predominantly neuroleptic induced to largely lithium induced.

These findings and interpretations were confirmed and amplified more recently in reviews by Goldman (1996a, 1996b). Goldman used the Food and Drug Administration Spontaneous Reporting System and a review of the published literature to identify 237 cases of neurotoxicity associated with lithium alone and lithium in combination with haloperidol or other neuroleptics. Several interesting findings emerged from this analysis: 1) the correlation between median lithium levels and neurological sequelae in the lithium and lithium-neuroleptic (other than haloperidol) groups was significant; 2) the prevalence of muscle rigidity and median neuroleptic doses were highest in the lithium-haloperidol group; 3) the occurrence of rigidity was similar in the lithium and lithium-neuroleptic groups; and 4) the diagnosis of definite or probable NMS with published criteria ranged up to 61% in the lithium-haloperidol group, significantly higher than in the lithium or the lithium-neuroleptic groups. Although these data provide support for the bipartate conceptualization of lithium-neuroleptic neurotoxicity proposal by Spring and Frankel (1981), the heterogeneity and overlap of cases led Goldman also to support the notion of a spectrum of neurotoxicity, ranging from neuroleptic induced (NMS) to primarily lithium induced.

Pathogenesis

Clinical reports of neurotoxicity have stimulated the development of experimental strategies designed to investigate potential interactions between lithium and neuroleptics. To date, there is no evidence of an interaction between neuroleptics and lithium on thermoregulation in animals (Clark and Lipton 1984). However, Shimomura et al. (1979) reported that a fatal hyperthermic reaction occurring after tranylcypromine administration in rats pretreated with lithium was inhibited by neuroleptics and possibly mediated by dopamine and serotonin. Some studies have detected direct pharmacokinetic interactions between these agents, resulting in altered plasma levels (Jefferson and Greist 1980; Nemes et al. 1987; Rivera-Calimlin et al. 1978). However, other investigators have found no pharmacokinetic interactions between lithium and neuroleptics (Demetriou et al. 1979; Forsman and Ohman 1977; D.F. Smith et al. 1977). Secondary metabolic changes resulting from toxicity due to one drug (e.g., dehydration in NMS) could alter the absorption and excretion of the other. For example, patients developing NMS while taking lithium may be at risk for developing lithium toxicity. This may occur because dehydration resulting from decreased fluid intake, sweating, and hyperthermia, and renal failure resulting from volume depletion and rhabdomyolysis, may elevate serum concentrations of lithium. In addition, other manifestations of NMS, such as hypoxia and hyperthermia, which may cause brain damage, could act synergistically with lithium in the destruction of neural tissue.

Data relevant to the problem of lithium-neuroleptic interactions also have been obtained from studies of the influence of neuroleptics on intracellular lithium levels. Some evidence shows that red blood cell (RBC) lithium levels correlate more closely with side effects than do plasma levels (Elizur et al. 1972; Hewick and Murray 1976). Several investigators reported that combined treatment results in increased RBC levels and tissue retention of lithium (Elizur et al. 1977; Strayhorn and Nash 1977). Pandey et al. (1979) and Ostrow et al. (1980) reported in vitro that phenothiazines, but not antidepressants or haloperidol, resulted in increased intracellular concentrations of lithium. Their data further suggest that cellular accumulation of lithium appeared to be caused by enhanced transport of lithium through passive leak diffusion. These findings were supported in a clinical study by von Knorring et al. (1982) in which patients taking a combination of neuroleptics and lithium had significantly higher RBC–to–plasma lithium ratios than did patients taking lithium alone. As in the study by Pandey et al. (1979), haloperidol did not have the same effect as phenothiazines or thioxanthenes. Thus, data on cellular transport of lithium provide a mechanism whereby combined therapy would augment lithium neurotoxicity, assuming RBC transport processes resemble those in neural tissue. This would explain cases of combined neurotoxicity involving phenothiazines in which acute effects of lithium and their sequelae predominate, consistent with the proposal advanced by Spring and Frankel (1981) that some of the reported cases represent lithium neurotoxicity primarily.

However, these effects have not been found in all studies. Ghadirian et al. (1989) found that haloperidol and chlorpromazine resulted in significantly lower RBC concentrations of lithium and lithium plasma ratios. In addition, these mechanisms (i.e., enhanced intracellular transport of lithium) seem less relevant in clarifying the pathophysiology underlying cases in which hyperthermia and extrapyramidal symptoms predominate, particularly when associated with haloperidol. However, analogous to experiments focusing on lithium transport, Nemes et al. (1987) reported that concurrent lithium administration resulted in higher concentrations of haloperidol in RBCs, plasma, and brain compared with administration of haloperidol alone. It is less clear whether these higher neuroleptic concentrations correlate with toxicity.

Although specific mechanisms have not been elucidated, it seems reasonable to propose that adverse effects of lithium-neuroleptic combinations on the extrapyramidal system reflect synergistic actions on dopamine neurotransmission (Bunney and Garland-Bunney 1987). Engel and Berggren (1980) reported that lithium has neuroleptic-like effects, possibly through inhibition of presynaptic catecholamine synthesis. Flemenbaum

(1977) reported that lithium, acting on both pre- and postsynaptic neurons, could inhibit behavior in rats that developed following administration of dopamine agonists. Reports of increased levels of dopamine metabolites in striatal but not other brain regions of rats chronically treated with lithium suggest enhancement of dopamine turnover or release (Eroglu et al. 1981; Fadda et al. 1980; Hesketh et al. 1978; Maggi and Enna 1980). Other investigators have shown that administration of lithium produces no changes in (Reches et al. 1984) or decreases (E. Friedman and Gershon 1973) dopamine metabolites in the striatum. In a retrospective clinical study of eight patients with mood disorders, Linnoila et al. (1983) found that lithium appeared to decrease dopamine and its metabolites in all patients.

More recently, Bowers et al. (1992) showed that the addition of lithium to perphenazine in the treatment of psychosis in 10 patients resulted in the blunting of the decline in plasma HVA observed in 13 patients treated with perphenazine alone. Bowers et al. (1992) noted that their findings were similar to earlier findings by Sternberg et al. (1983), in which the expected decline in cerebrospinal fluid HVA was not observed in patients treated with lithium in combination with haloperidol. These reports suggest that lithium may interfere with compensatory depolarization inactivation of dopamine systems in response to neuroleptic treatment.

In studies of chronic lithium administration in animals, no effect of lithium was found on haloperidol-induced increases in dopamine metabolism in the striatum, nucleus accumbens, or frontal cortex (Meller and Friedman 1981; Reches et al. 1984). However, substantial evidence suggests that lithium prevents the development of behavioral manifestations of neuroleptic-induced supersensitivity of dopamine receptors (Bunney and Garland-Bunney 1987). Studies of dopamine receptor binding in rat brain that used [^{3}H]-spiroperidol suggested that lithium may block the development of supersensitivity in some dopamine pathways by inhibiting the increase in number of dopamine receptors (Pert et al. 1978; Rosenblatt et al. 1980), although not all studies have successfully replicated this finding (Bloom et al. 1983; Lal et al. 1978; Pittman et al. 1984; Reches et al. 1982; Staunton et al. 1982a, 1982b). Conceivably, lithium-induced inhibition of compensatory changes in dopamine receptor function could augment neuroleptic dopamine receptor blockade and increase the likelihood of neurotoxicity, at least during chronic treatment. However, the acute effects of lithium on dopamine transmission and on neuroleptic-induced changes in dopamine activity appear to be variable and therefore difficult to reconcile with a consistent mechanism for understanding combined neurotoxicity.

Because administration of lithium alters several other neurotransmitter systems, especially enhancing serotoninergic activity (Blier et al. 1987), it may be worthwhile to consider the effects of these neurotransmitters in producing synergistic toxicity when lithium is combined with neuroleptics (Bunney and Garland-Bunney 1987).

Studies of neurotransmitter and receptor function have been inconclusive; however, potential synergistic interactions of lithium and neuroleptics on intracellular mechanisms involving secondary messengers also merit consideration. For example, lithium has been shown in some studies to inhibit dopamine-sensitive adenylate cyclase in the caudate nucleus of the rat (Bunney and Garland-Bunney 1987). Geisler and Klysner (1977) found that inhibition of dopamine-sensitive adenylate cyclase in rat striatum was significantly enhanced when flupenthixol and lithium were combined as compared with when either agent was used alone.

In addition, increased recognition of the role of phosphoinositide metabolism in receptor mechanism and transmembrane signaling suggests that this system may be worth examining in relation to combined neurotoxicity (Rasmussen 1986a, 1986b; Snider et al. 1987). It has been firmly established that lithium, at concentrations comparable to therapeutic levels, inhibits *myo*-inositol-1-phosphatase, resulting in significantly lower *myo*-inositol and raised inositol-1-phosphate levels in the brain (Sherman et al. 1985). Although it is unclear whether this effect persists with chronic lithium treatment (Renshaw et al. 1986a, 1986b; Sherman et al. 1985), a reduced ability to form *myo*-inositol could seriously compromise neurotransmitter systems that depend on phosphoinositide metabolism (Renshaw et al. 1986a; Snider et al. 1987).

Furthermore, investigations of the phosphoinositide system may be relevant because phenothiazines have been reported to stimulate or partially inhibit phospholipase C, depending on dosage, albeit in the micromolar range compared with nanomolar clinical levels (Walenga et al. 1981). Phospholipase C mediates the hydrolysis of inositol phosphate to diacylglycerol and inositol-1,2,5-triphosphate in response to extracellular receptor agonists (Rasmussen 1986a, 1986b). Thus, coadministration of lithium and neuroleptics could result in synergistic effects on this messenger system, thereby altering neurotransmitter-stimulated calcium-dependent metabolic processes and augmenting toxic effects of either agent.

In summary, the question of synergy raised by W.J. Cohen and Cohen in 1974 remains enigmatic and unresolved. There clearly have been rare but definite cases of a severe encephalopathic syndrome, sometimes with persistent neurological damage, that has developed in patients taking lithium in combination with neuroleptics. These cases appear to represent a continuum of neurotoxicity, ranging from cases resembling lithium neurotoxicity to cases indistinguishable from NMS. Most studies of sample populations of patients treated with this combination attest to the rarity of this reaction and suggest that if synergy occurs between these drugs, it occurs only under unusual circumstances in certain predisposed individuals. The effect of the introduction of atypical antipsychotics on this interaction remains to be determined. Laboratory studies support a mechanism whereby phenothiazine neuroleptics may facilitate the influx of lithium intracellularly and enhance the neurotoxicity of lithium. In contrast, no consistent action of lithium on dopaminergic or other neurotransmitter or second messenger systems has emerged that correlates with enhanced extrapyramidal effects of neuroleptics in the presence of lithium or with the possibility that combined therapy with lithium may enhance the risk or severity of NMS-like hyperthermic reactions.

🖅 Sympathomimetic Drugs

Amphetamines

The clinical and pathological features of toxicity with central nervous system (CNS) stimulants have been described in detail (Clark and Lipton 1984; Fischman 1987). Administration of toxic doses of amphetamines and related drugs leads to a characteristic syndrome consisting of sweating, mydriasis, tachycardia, hyperactivity, and confusion, which may progress to hyperthermia, delirium, seizures, arrhythmias, shock, renal failure, DIC, and death. Because of the prevalence of abuse of these drugs, it is important to be aware of the clinical manifestations of toxicity and to contrast this presentation with NMS and disorders associated with other psychotropic agents. In addition, investigation of amphetamine toxicity may provide a broader picture of pharmacological mechanisms underlying hyperthermic syndromes in general.

Hyperthermia is often found in relation to severe amphetamine toxicity (Clark and Lipton 1984; E.M. Sellers et al. 1979). As reviewed by Clark and Lipton (1984), amphetamine-induced hyperthermia appears to reflect enhanced heat production in skeletal muscle. In support of this, fatal amphetamine-induced hyperthermia in dogs can be blocked by curare (Zalis et al. 1965). Increased heat production in skeletal muscle usually results from hyperactivity, agitation, or seizures. Increases in serum CPK and elevations in body temperature have been reported in the aftermath of convulsive activity (Belton et al. 1967; Wachtel et al. 1987). Although increased motor activity caused by locomotor stimulation or convulsions is typical, and probably accounts for heat production in most cases, some patients develop NMS-like syndromes characterized by extreme muscle rigidity. The development of rigidity may be centrally mediated, or rigidity may develop secondary to the loss of control of calcium-dependent contractile mechanisms in skeletal muscle as a result of excessive rise in muscle temperature (Fuchs 1975).

Some investigators (W.M. Davis et al. 1974; E.M. Sellers et al. 1979) have recommended use of neuroleptics to treat severe hyperthermic reactions associated with amphetamine toxicity, reasoning that neuroleptics may reduce agitation and possibly reverse amphetamine-induced peripheral α-adrenergic activation and vasoconstriction. Although neuroleptics could prevent decompensation in an agitated patient, the tendency of neuroleptics to impair the thermoregulatory response to a heat load, to increase heat production through rigidity, and to reduce heat loss by peripheral inhibition of sweating could override potential beneficial effects once hyperthermia supervened (Kosten and Kleber 1987). Chlorpromazine was administered to two patients reviewed by E.M. Sellers et al. (1979); one died shortly after treatment began, and the other survived but became obtunded and hypotensive after administration of chlorpromazine (Ginsberg et al. 1970). In contrast, Gary and Saidi (1978) reported the effective use of intravenous droperidol in treating a patient who developed a temperature of 42°C following methamphetamine intoxication.

3,4-Methylenedioxymethamphetamine (MDMA)

MDMA and other methylenedioxy analogues of amphetamine have received increasing attention in connection with the metabolic consequences of their abuse, as reviewed by several investigators (Gill et al. 2002; Gold et al. 2001; Green et al. 1995; Hegadoren et al. 1999; J.A. Henry 2000) and discussed in Chapter 3. These drugs appear to have some resemblance to hallucinogenic drugs as well as the sympathomimetic stimulant effects of amphetamine. However, MDMA has only one-tenth the stimulant effect of amphetamine and is also a potent releaser of serotonin as well as an inhibitor of its uptake (Green et al. 1995; McKenna and Peroutka 1990; P.D. Mueller and Korey 1998; Rudnick and Wall 1992; S.R. White et al. 1996).

Consistent with CNS stimulants, MDMA has been associated with the entire range of NMS-like symptoms in clinical case reports (Gowing et al. 2002). This has included hyperthermia, hypertonicity, rhabdomyolysis, and autonomic changes leading to renal or respiratory failure, DIC, and death in some cases. However, the situation with MDMA is more complex. First, the development of hyperthermic toxicity has not been dose related (Gill et al. 2002; Hegadoren et al. 1999). In addition, the incidence of hyperthermic deaths attributable to MDMA was found to be less in New York City compared with reports from the United Kingdom (Gill et al. 2002). These disparities have been attributed to the contributory role of overexertion in hot settings during "rave" dances, which may have been more common in the United Kingdom. Hyperthermic NMS-like states may develop following MDMA abuse primarily in association with stimulant-driven dehydration and exertional heatstroke (Green et al. 1995). Another distinguishing feature of MDMA toxicity is its resemblance to serotonin syndrome (Green et al. 1995; Hegadoren et al. 1999; P.D. Mueller and Korey 1998), which is consistent with its pronounced acute effects on serotonin (Chapter 3).

The treatment of toxic reactions and hyperthermia secondary to MDMA ingestion is generally supportive and empirical. Ventilatory assistance, cooling measures, anticonvulsants, and fluid replacement are recommended. The use of dantrolene was beneficial in a few cases (Green et al. 1995; Murthy et al. 1997; Singarajah and Lavies 1992a, 1992b) but remains unproven and controversial (Hegadoren et al. 1999; Watson et al. 1993).

Cocaine

Hyperthermia appears to play a major role in fatal cocaine intoxication (Callaway and Clark 1994; Catravas and Waters 1981; Crandall et al. 2002; Daras et al. 1995; J.A. Henry 2000; Loghmanee and Tobak 1986; Olson and Benowitz 1987; Tanvetyanon et al. 2001). Cases have been reported in which the intravenous, intranasal, inhalational, or oral administration of cocaine resulted in hyperthermia associated with seizures, agitation, mutism, rhabdomyolysis, and renal, respiratory, or cardiovascular failure (Bettinger 1980; Krohn et al. 1988; Merigian and Roberts 1987; J.R. Roberts et al. 1984).

The association between cocaine intoxication and acute rhabdomyolysis apart from hyperthermia has been emphasized (D. Roth et al. 1988). D. Roth et al. (1988) reviewed 39 patients who presented with rhabdomyolysis after cocaine intoxication. These patients typically presented with agitation and myalgias. Sixty-two percent of the patients had temperatures above 38°C, and 33% had temperatures above 40°C. Death was most likely to occur in patients with rhabdomyolysis who developed acute renal failure, liver dysfunction, and DIC. Myonecrosis in these patients may result from the vasoconstrictive and ischemic effects of cocaine or by a direct toxic effect on muscle metabolism (Herzlich et al. 1988; Venkatachari et al. 1988). Similarly, Daras et al. (1995) reported on 14 patients who presented with rhabdomyolysis after cocaine use. All but one had concomitant hyperthermia, but fewer than half presented with muscle rigidity. Five (35.7%) patients died of renal failure or cardiorespiratory arrest.

Hyperthermia associated with cocaine probably results from multiple factors, including increased heat production resulting from muscular activity and seizures, compounded by reduced heat dissipation due to vasoconstriction (Crandall et al. 2002; Olson and Benowitz 1987). Catravas and Waters (1981) reported that neuromuscular blockade by pancuronium effectively antagonized cocaine-induced hyperthermia in dogs. They also showed that hyperthermia could be blocked by hypothermia and chlorpromazine. Although the use of neuroleptics has been suggested in the treatment of cocaine poisoning (Olson and Benowitz 1987), their efficacy may relate to nonspecific sedation because the potent dopamine receptor antagonist pimozide, unlike chlorpromazine, had no effect in preventing lethality from cocaine in dogs (Catravas and Waters 1981).

Considering the clinical resemblance between some cases of cocaine intoxication and NMS, Kosten and Kleber (1987, 1988) proposed that rapid death in cocaine abusers represents a variant of NMS. They speculated that hyperthermia in cocaine abusers results from a relative decline in postsynaptic dopamine availability in hypothalamic and mesolimbic systems following a period of sustained dopamine stimulation during active cocaine use. Based on this hypothesis, Kosten and Kleber (1988) suggested that dopamine antagonists may be contraindicated in cocaine overdose and, conversely, that dopamine agonists may reverse this potentially fatal syndrome.

The resemblance and association between cocaine-induced hyperthermia and NMS have been echoed by subsequent investigators (Daras et al. 1995; Tanvetyanon et al. 2001). For example, a higher incidence of NMS has been reported among cocaine abusers receiving neuroleptics (5.1%) than among nonabusers (0.2%) (Akpaffiong and Ruiz 1991). However, there are differences between the syndromes in the dissociation of component symptoms. Cocaine abuse is associated with hyperthermia in the context of high ambient temperature (Marzuk et al. 1998) and frequently in the absence of muscle rigidity (Daras et al. 1995). Systemic hyperthermia is commonly preceded and accompanied by an agitated delirium following cocaine use, whereas the mental status in NMS is characteristically akinetic mutism, or catatonia, which is a rare finding in cocaine abusers (Gingrich et al. 1998).

Fenfluramine

von Muhlendahl and Krienke (1979) published a review of toxicity due to fenfluramine, an amphetamine derivative used as an anorexic agent and in the treatment of autism. Their findings may apply to other derivatives of fenfluramine as well. They reviewed 53 case reports of fenfluramine intoxication and found that hypertoxicity, rigor, trismus, and opisthotonus were reported in 34% of cases, tachycardia was seen in 81%, sweating was frequently observed, and hyperthermia (37.6°C to 42.8°C) was seen in 25%

of cases. In addition to hyperthermia, coma, and convulsions, the signs of nystagmus, hypertonia, trismus, hyperreflexia, excitation, and sweating characterized the clinical syndrome of fenfluramine intoxication. Three patients with temperature above 40°C died. In one case, high plasma levels of intracellular enzymes detected 2 hours after drug ingestion were suggestive of muscle necrosis. Signs of intoxication occurred 30–60 minutes after ingestion and lasted several days, although in 90% of the lethal cases, cardiac arrest and death occurred within 1–4 hours after ingestion.

Manifestations of fenfluramine toxicity may reflect abnormalities in serotoninergic mechanisms and represent a form of serotonin syndrome (Chapter 3). Fenfluramine produces rapid release and inhibition of uptake of serotonin, resulting in long-term depletion of serotonin stores (Schuster et al. 1986; Sulpizio et al. 1978). Sulpizio et al. (1978) tested a variety of pharmacological agents on fenfluramine-induced hyperthermia produced in rats maintained in a warm environment (25°C to 28°C). They concluded that hyperthermia results from increased serotonin from presynaptic stores because the hyperthermic response to fenfluramine was abolished by pretreatment with parachlorophenylalanine, cyproheptadine, and methysergide. In addition, they found that neuroleptics varied in the ability to antagonize fenfluramine-induced hyperthermia. Potent dopamine receptor blockers, such as pimozide and haloperidol, were inactive or enhanced hyperthermia, whereas less potent neuroleptics had a variable effect or, in the case of clozapine, completely antagonized the hyperthermic response. This effect of clozapine suggested to these investigators that clozapine has significant antiserotoninergic effects and may act to preserve a balance of dopamine and serotonin in the brain.

In contrast to the variable effects of neuroleptics on fenfluramine-induced hyperthermia reported by Sulpizio et al. (1978), von Muhlendahl and Krienke (1979) cited studies on experimental amphetamine intoxication in animals (W.M. Davis et al. 1974) as a basis for suggesting that neuroleptics and adrenergic antagonists may be useful in treating fenfluramine toxicity.

Pathogenesis

In animals, amphetamines generally elevate body temperature, although this effect is variable and depends on experimental factors (including the species chosen for study and ambient temperature). Although substantial evidence implicates central dopamine pathways in the hypothermic response to amphetamines administered in a cold environment (T.F. Lee et al. 1985) (see Chapter 2), the mechanisms underlying the hyperthermic response remain uncertain. Amphetamines may produce a peripheral thermogenic effect caused by release of systemic catecholamines (Weis 1973; Zalis et al. 1967), which may be compounded by adrenergic-mediated inhibition of heat loss caused by vasoconstriction (Clark and Lipton 1984). As discussed earlier, clinical and animal data suggest that stimulant-induced hyperthermia also may be a result of increased heat production by skeletal muscle associated with hyperactivity, agitation, seizures, or rigidity. Rhabdomyolysis, which is frequently observed in relation to hyperthermia in these cases, also may reflect multiple determinants, including exertion and rigidity of muscle, heat effects, ischemia, and direct myotoxic effects of stimulants (Daras et al. 1995).

However, an additional site of amphetamine action in triggering a hyperthermic reaction may be central; hyperthermia can be induced by cerebral ventricular injection and blocked by intraventricular administration of 6-hydroxydopamine (Clark and Lipton 1984). Furthermore, because α- and β-adrenergic antagonists inhibit and tricyclic antidepressants enhance amphetamine-induced hyperthermia, this response may be mediated by the action of amphetamines in releasing norepinephrine. As noted by Clark and Lipton (1984), central administration of norepinephrine generally lowers body temperature in primates and other species, which reinforces the notion that the hyperthermic response to amphetamines may be due primarily to norepinephrine stimulation of motor activity rather than direct norepinephrine effects on central thermoregulatory mechanisms. However, Wirtshafter et al. (1978) reported that in rats maintained at room temperature, electrolytic lesions of the nucleus accumbens and olfactory tubercle antagonized amphetamine-induced hyperthermia but did not block amphetamine-induced hyperactivity. Similarly, Norman et al. (1987) and other investigators (Feigenbaum and Yanai 1985; Grahame-Smith 1971) found a dose-related dissociation between behavioral stimulation and hyperthermia in rats following amphetamine administration. Thus, the hyperthermic response to amphetamines may reflect direct effects on central thermoregulatory processes in addition to nonspecific changes in motor activity.

Amphetamines and related sympathomimetic drugs affect monoamine neurotransmitters other than norepinephrine, which may be implicated in the production of hyperthermia. In particular, significant increases in serotonin activity appear to account convincingly for the development of hyperthermia and a form of the serotonin syndrome caused by fenfluramine and methylenedioxy analogues of amphetamine (Gill et al. 2002; Green et al. 1995; Hegadoren et al. 1999; P.D. Mueller and Korey 1998; S.R. White et al. 1996) (see Chapter 3).

Moreover, the reinforcing and stimulant properties of these drugs appear to be related to an increase in dopamine activity resulting from potentiation of release and inhibition of reuptake of this neurotransmitter (Callaway and Clark 1994; Fischman 1987; T.F. Lee et al. 1985). Implication of dopamine in amphetamine-induced hyperthermia is suggested by studies in which hyperthermia was blocked by electrolytic lesions of the mesolimbic dopamine system (Wirtshafter et al. 1978) or by administration of dopamine antagonists or dopamine-depleting drugs (Ulus et al. 1975). In addition, Norman et al. (1987) reported that short-term pretreatment with neuroleptics resulted in increased sensitivity to the hyperthermic effects of amphetamine in rats studied at room temperature, perhaps reflecting the development of supersensitivity of dopamine receptors.

However, data suggesting the involvement of dopamine in amphetamine-induced hyperthermia conflict with evidence supporting the role of dopamine in mediating pathways that subserve heat dissipation and the development of hypothermia (T.F. Lee et al. 1985) (see Chapter 2). Perhaps the hyperthermic response is mediated primarily by norepinephrine derived from excessive dopamine (Przewlocka and Kaluza 1973). Otherwise, differences among studies in the dopamine-mediated effects of amphetamines on temperature may be due to differences in experimental procedures, including species differences, duration, dose, route, and localization of drug administration and ambient temperature (T.F. Lee et al. 1985).

Alternatively, the development of hyperthermia, rather than hypothermia, as a result of dopamine-mediated amphetamine effects may depend on the state of or changes in dopamine receptor sensitivity, different classes of dopamine receptors, reciprocal or feedback interactions between dopamine pathways, or the influence of dopamine on other neurotransmitter systems. For example, based on studies in which apomorphine, amphetamine, and dopamine produced hyperthermic reactions in rodents pretreated with haloperidol, reserpine, and serotonin antagonists, S. Yamawaki et al. (1983) and others (Feigenbaum and Yanai 1985; Fjalland 1979; Frey 1975) proposed that dopaminergic agonists may activate two separate dopamine-related thermoregulatory pathways in the brain, one resulting in hypothermia and the other in hyperthermia. S. Yamawaki et al. (1983) further proposed that the latter mechanism is mediated by secondary activation of serotonin and is haloperidol insensitive. Although this model is highly speculative, it implies that under certain circumstances, amphetamines could preferentially activate a dopamine- or serotonin-mediated hyperthermic pathway that could be blocked by serotonin antagonists and enhanced by neuroleptic blockade of the haloperidol-sensitive dopamine hypothermia mechanism (Sulpizio et al. 1978).

Although central mechanisms underlying amphetamine-induced hyperthermia remain speculative and complex, it may be worthwhile to compare this condition with other hyperthermic disorders. In particular, it is tempting to consider hyperthermia due to amphetamines as a pharmacological model for "functional" cases of malignant catatonia (see Chapter 5). As discussed earlier, clinical features and animal data strongly support the similarities between serotonin syndrome and acute toxicity associated with MDMA and fenfluramine. In contrast, any relation between amphetamine-induced hyperthermia and NMS is unclear and problematic. Some investigators have suggested that the pathophysiological response to the enhancement of dopamine activity by amphetamine-like drugs may be a useful model for investigating mechanisms underlying NMS (Kosten and Kleber 1987, 1988; Norman et al. 1987). Acute treatment with neuroleptics results in a short-term, compensatory increase in dopamine synthesis, release, and turnover. Before the development of depolarization inactivation with chronic neuroleptic treatment, this may correlate with the onset of NMS symptoms during the initial phases of neuroleptic treatment. Accordingly, NMS may resemble acute dystonic reactions. Excessive dopamine activity has been implicated in the etiology of neuroleptic-induced dystonic movements (Tarsy 1983). However, pharmacological mechanisms underlying dystonia and NMS appear to be different because NMS responds to dopamine agonists and is relatively refractory to anticholinergic drugs. Furthermore, enhancement of dopamine activity cannot explain the development of NMS-like conditions in patients deprived of dopamine agonists in Parkinson's disease.

Although dopamine overactivity in NMS seems unlikely, amphetamine-like effects may relate to the proposal of Schibuk and Schachter (1986) that NMS may result from excessive norepinephrine relative to dopamine activity. Similarly, Ansseau et al. (1986) suggested that NMS may result from an interaction between norepinephrine and dopamine systems. Finally, peripheral catecholamines may be significantly elevated in NMS and may contribute to the generation of heat (Feibel and Schiffer 1981), as proposed for amphetamine intoxication by some investigators (Weis 1973; Zalis et al. 1967).

Psychedelic Drugs

Phencyclidine

Phencyclidine (PCP) was initially introduced as an anesthetic, but following reports of postanesthetic psychotic states, pronounced muscle rigidity, and seizure activity, it ceased to be marketed in the United States. Nevertheless, since the 1960s, PCP has continued to be used as a drug of abuse and appears to be a unique psychoactive drug with diverse neurobehavioral effects, including depressant, stimulant, hallucinogenic, and analgesic properties.

Signs of PCP intoxication are dose related. At low doses, patients may show ataxia, slurred speech, numbness of the extremities, sweating, muscle rigidity, and signs of catatonia. Catatonic features, including staring and mutism, are characteristic of PCP and may account for the "dissociative" state or "sensory blockade" that has been described, similar to neuroleptic analgesia. At higher doses of PCP, anesthesia, stupor, and coma may appear, accompanied by elevated heart rate and blood pressure, hypersalivation, sweating, fever, and convulsions.

In a review of more than 250 cases of PCP overdose, Rappolt et al. (1979) divided intoxication into three stages:

1. In stage I (serum concentration=25–90 ng/mL), patients showed nystagmus, hyperreflexia, generalized spasticity, salivation, ataxia, myoclonus, and behavioral toxicity ranging from catatonic stupor, hallucinations, and disorientation to combativeness and violence. Diuresis, acidification of the urine, and treatment with diazepam and propranolol were recommended during this stage.
2. In stage II (serum concentration=100–300 ng/mL), patients became stuporous and verbally unresponsive and developed hypertensive and tachycardic episodes.
3. In stage III (serum concentration>300 ng/mL), patients were generally comatose. In addition to tachycardia and hypertension, tachypnea developed with the potential for apnea. "Boardlike" muscle rigidity, myoclonus, opisthotonus, and seizures occurred.

In stages II and III, a potentially life-threatening "adrenergic crisis" or "dopaminergic storm" sometimes appeared in 72–96 hours after drug ingestion. This manifested as a hypertensive encephalopathy or "malignant-type" hyperthermia. Rappolt et al. (1979) advocated use of propranolol to prevent this from occurring.

McCarron et al. (1981a, 1981b) reported the results of an extensive survey of 1,000 cases of PCP intoxication. In agreement with the results of Barton et al. (1981), they found that behavioral abnormalities, nystagmus, and hypertension were the most common manifestations of acute PCP intoxication. Violent and agitated behavior was more commonly observed than lethargy and stupor. Hypothermia (6.4%) was more than twice as common as hyperthermia (2.6%). Rhabdomyolysis, occasionally associated with renal failure, was the most common serious medical complication of acute PCP intoxication (Barton et al. 1981). Serum CPK was greater than 300 IU in 70% of the patients in which it was tested. Patients with elevated CPK were equally likely to be violent, agitated, or calm. The highest CPK was more than 400,000 IU. McCarron et al. (1981a) divided neuropsychiatric manifestations of PCP intoxication into four major (coma, catatonia, toxic psychosis, acute brain syndrome) and five minor (lethargy, bizarre behavior, violence, agitation, euphoria) patterns. Among patients with coma, 50% showed generalized rigidity, 25% had hypothermia, and 8% had hyperthermia above 38.9°C.

The clinical picture of PCP toxicity emerging from smaller series of cases is less consistent, with varying reports of hyperthermia, rigidity, and rhabdomyolysis (Clark and Lipton 1984). Armen et al. (1984) reported three cases, one fatal, in which PCP intoxication resulted in agitation and combative behavior, severe hyperthermia (41.7°C to 42.2°C), respiratory failure, and coma. All three patients had rhabdomyolysis and severe liver necrosis. The investigators compared these reactions with malignant hyperthermia of anesthesia and speculated that the marked temperature elevations could be related to the anesthetic properties of PCP. Consistent with this notion, ketamine, a related arylcyclohexylamine anesthetic, also has been associated with hyperthermia intraoperatively in patients with known susceptibility to malignant hyperthermia (Page et al. 1972; Roervik and Stovner 1974). This suggests that hyperthermia associated with arylcyclohexylamines may share some features with mechanisms underlying malignant hyperthermia.

Cogen et al. (1978) described two patients who developed PCP-associated acute rhabdomyolysis. They concluded that muscle necrosis was directly related to dystonia and excessive motor activity in these patients. They cited evidence from Kuncl and Meltzer (1974), which indicated that denervation of motor nerve input prevented muscle damage in PCP-treated restrained rats. However, further work by the same group has shown that the PCP-restrained experimental myopathy also could be inhibited by adrenalectomy, adrenal demedullation, treatment with β-adrenergic antagonists, and pretreatment with dantrolene (Ross-Canada et al. 1983). Furthermore, dantrolene diminished muscle damage but did not reduce locomotor activity or stereotyped behavior observed in rats treated with PCP. Thus, the rhabdomyolytic effect of PCP may be multidetermined and dependent on catecholamine stimulation as well as motor nerve activity, both of which may contribute to muscle damage through the release of calcium in the sarcoplasmic reticulum (Ross-Canada et al. 1983).

Pathogenesis

Hyperthermia or hypothermia in cases of PCP intoxication may be multifactorial in origin. Hyperthemia may be related to seizures (Wachtel et al. 1987) or to the frenetic overactivity and combativeness of patients subjected to the sympathomimetic or stimulant properties of PCP. PCP has a propensity to affect muscle, resulting in heat generation and necrosis, possibly mediated by motor nerve activity, peripheral catecholamines, or more direct myotoxic effects of the drug (Meltzer et al. 1972; Ross-Canada et al. 1983). PCP increases oxygen consumption in rats in vivo, increases mitochondrial oxygen consumption in rat liver homogenates (Domino 1964), and appears to uncouple oxidative phosphorylation (Lees 1961), all of which may contribute to the peripheral generation of heat.

The central neurochemical basis of behavioral and thermoregulatory changes associated with PCP intoxication is unknown. PCP affects several neurotransmitter systems; it antagonizes excitatory amino acids, enhances noradrenergic and possibly serotoninergic activity, possesses anticholinergic properties, and binds to a specific PCP receptor that is shared with psychotomimetic benzomorphan opioids (Balster 1987). The anticholinergic properties of PCP may impair heat loss and contribute to hyperthermia, but other pharmacological properties of PCP may play a role in thermoregulatory disorders associated with PCP and related drugs.

PCP has amphetamine-like behavioral properties and has been characterized as an indirect dopamine agonist. PCP has been reported to inhibit dopamine reuptake, facilitate its release, and secondarily affect dopamine synthesis and metabolism (Balster 1987; T.S. Rao et al. 1989). However, as in the case of amphetamines, it is difficult to relate enhancement of dopamine activity with the clinical development of hyperthermia, rigidity, and rhabdomyolysis, apart from drug effects on locomotor activity. In contrast, the dopamine agonist properties of PCP could be invoked to explain the more common development of hypothermia in patients intoxicated with PCP (T.F. Lee et al. 1985).

Although PCP toxicity may present as an NMS-like syndrome composed of hyperthermia, sympathetic activation, rhabdomyolysis, and striking muscle rigidity, the unique behavioral and pharmacological properties of the drug may represent an intriguing pharmacological model for exploring potential mechanisms underlying malignant catatonia due to the major psychoses (Rappolt et al. 1979).

Lysergic Acid Diethylamide (LSD)

Interestingly, LSD, a psychotomimetic drug with pharmacological effects similar to those of serotonin, produces hyperthermia along with other sympathomimetic effects in humans and animal species (Clark and Lipton 1984; Domino 1964; Gorodetzky and Isbell 1964). For example, Klock et al. (1973) reported eight patients who developed hyperactivity, psychosis, and sympathetic activation leading to coagulopathy, respiratory arrest, and coma. One patient presented with dystonia, and four patients developed elevated temperature (38.2°C to 41.7°C). S.A. Friedman and Hirsch (1971) reported a patient with a temperature of 41.3°C, associated with psychosis and hyperactivity. Although hyperthermia in these cases may reflect extreme exertion, it also underscores the potential significance of central serotoninergic mechanisms underlying hyperthermic reactions (Frey 1975; Glennon 1990; Jacobs 1976; S. Yamawaki et al. 1983).

Although LSD intoxication may reflect a variant of the serotonin syndrome, Bakkert et al. (1990) described a case including coma, rigidity, and rhabdomyolysis, which they considered identical to NMS. Perera et al. (1995) reported a case of incipient catatonia and psychosis after LSD ingestion, which progressed to catatonic stupor after treatment with haloperidol.

🗟 Anticholinergic Drugs

Several drugs used in clinical psychopharmacology possess significant anticholinergic activity. Antiparkinsonian agents and some antidepressant and antipsychotics act as muscarinic antagonists and may elevate body temperature either as a result of inhibition of cholinergic activity within the central thermoregulatory centers (Lin et al. 1980; Torline 1992) or as a result of interference with peripheral heat loss by inhibiting sweating (Baldessarini 1985; Caroff et al. 2000b; Knochel 1989; Knochel and Reed 1994). In fact, use of atropine and related agents has been associated with compromise of thermoregulation in hot environments (Clark and Lipton 1984; Cullumbine and Miles 1956) and are considered as risk factors for heatstroke (see Chapter 2). However, in some experimental studies of the effects of atropine in healthy subjects exercising or exposed to heat, body temperature did not rise to dangerous levels. Inhibition of sweating was no more than 50%, resulting in only partial impairment of heat-loss mechanisms. This led Clark and Lipton (1984) to conclude that therapeutic doses of atropine are not likely to cause significant hyperthermia, at least in healthy subjects in thermally neutral environments, and that in order for hyperthermia to develop in patients, overdosage and excessive heat load or further inhibition of heat loss perhaps through central mechanisms would be necessary. However, once sweating ceases after taking anticholinergic drugs in a hot environment, body temperature may rise precipitously even with moderate exercise by patients (Caroff et al. 2000b; Knochel 1989).

Intoxication with anticholinergic drugs results in a well-described syndrome of atropinic poisoning that is characterized by central and peripheral signs (e.g., dry mouth, flushed dry skin, dilated pupils, blurred vision, tachycardia, urinary retention, and intestinal paralysis), which may progress to ataxia, hyperactivity, agitation, increased muscle tone, delirium, and coma. In a survey of cases of anticholinergic poisoning, Shader and Greenblatt (1971) found temperatures above 37.7°C in 18% of adults and

25% of children. Temperatures above 40°C are less common (Clark and Lipton 1984). In the absence of external heat stress in these cases, Clark and Lipton (1984) speculated that agitation and delirium resulting from toxic doses may have contributed to hyperthermia by the endogenous generation of heat.

Because of the pronounced signs of anticholinergic toxicity in the periphery, the inhibition of sweating, and the uncommon appearance of severe temperature elevations, rhabdomyolysis, and rigidity, hyperthermia due to anticholinergic intoxication is unlikely to be mistaken for NMS. This is important because treatment may differ; physostigmine serves as a specific antidote in atropine poisoning but has no effect in NMS (Krull and Risse 1986; Patel and Bristow 1987; Torline 1992).

Anticholinergics are often used in psychiatry in combination with other agents, including neuroleptics and antidepressants. As a result, their inhibitory effect on sweating may contribute to the emergence of hyperthermia due to thermoregulatory effects of other drugs used concurrently. For example, up to 23% of cases of NMS developed when anticholinergic antiparkinsonian drugs were administered with neuroleptics (Kurlan et al. 1984), and nearly half of NMS cases involved treatment with either antiparkinsonian or tricyclic antidepressant agents (Levenson 1985). Thus, anticholinergics may contribute to heat stress when hyperthermia develops in association with neuroleptics or other drugs.

🐚 Conclusion

The clinical manifestations of NMS, including hyperthermia, rigidity, and autonomic and mental status changes, constitute a hypermetabolic syndrome that is not specific for this neuroleptic-induced disorder. These clinical features may be found in association with a broad range of systemic and local disorders affecting brain function. Diverse pharmacological agents, including various neuropsychiatric drugs, which may affect thermoregulation by a variety of proposed mechanisms, have been associated with NMS-like syndromes. Recognition of the nonspecificity of NMS symptoms and familiarity with the disease processes and drugs that have been associated with these symptoms are essential in the management of patients presenting with hyperthermic and hypermetabolic syndromes. In addition, examination of the spectrum of drugs associated with NMS-like conditions provides a rationale to expand investigations of the theoretical mechanisms underlying these disorders.

Numerous cases have now been reported in which abrupt withdrawal of dopamine agonists from patients treated for Parkinson's disease resulted in hyperthermic reactions indistinguishable from NMS. In addition to data on NMS-like reactions in patients treated with dopamine-depleting drugs or experiencing "freezing" episodes during levodopa administration, these reactions add clinical support to the hypothesis implicating hypodopaminergic activity as a primary mechanism underlying the development of NMS.

Although hyperthermia is not typical of lithium toxicity, lithium in combination with neuroleptics has clearly been associated with the development of NMS. Lithium, which has been shown to inhibit the development of behavioral supersensitivity following neuroleptic administration, also has serotoninergic properties and is increasingly recognized as having significant effects on second-messenger systems. Whether these or other pharmacological effects of lithium act in synergy with neuroleptics to enhance the toxicity of either agent remains an intriguing area of research.

Some sympathomimetic and psychedelic drugs, in cases of overdose, also have been associated with hyperthermia. Behavioral neurotoxicity resulting in hyperactivity, agitation, or convulsions is typical of these agents and appears to account for heat production, but NMS-like cases with rigidity and rhabdomyolysis also have been reported. The pharmacological profiles of drugs in these classes led to speculation that augmentation of dopamine, serotonin, or norepinephrine activity could be involved, although data to support this are contradictory and inconclusive. However, increasing data suggest that hyperthermia and neurotoxicity of MDMA and fenfluramine represent forms of the serotonin syndrome.

In contrast, anticholinergic drugs facilitate the development of hyperthermia by peripheral inhibition of sweating but are unlikely to produce typical NMS or serotonin syndrome symptoms when administered alone.

Contrasting effects of drugs on central neurotransmitter systems notwithstanding, NMS-like instances of drug toxicity have in common the activation of thermoregulatory effector mechanisms involved in the development of hypermetabolism and hyperthermia due to a variety of drugs and disease processes.

C H A P T E R 5

Malignant Catatonia

Hyperthermia was recognized historically as a potential life-threatening complication of acute psychotic illness. In the last half century, however, advances in psychopharmacology and medical care have enabled clinicians to effectively treat most psychotic disorders, so that inexorable progression to hyperthermia and death now appears less likely to occur. Paradoxically, as detailed in the previous chapters of this book, many of those very same psychotropic drugs that have dramatically improved the management of psychiatric conditions have themselves been associated with the development of uncommon but potentially fatal hyperthermic syndromes.

In 1832, Calmeil described a fulminating psychotic disorder characterized by mounting hyperthermia and extreme motor excitement, which progressed to stuporous exhaustion. In those cases ending in death, the paucity of findings on autopsy was puzzling and in sharp contrast to the catastrophic clinical manifestations. This disorder was subsequently reported by Luther Bell (1849) in his article published in *The American Journal of Insanity* and by numerous other American and foreign authors throughout the pre–antipsychotic drug era. The world literature of this period is replete with descriptions, proposed mechanisms, and names for this condition. Competing terminologies included *Bell's mania, mortal catatonia, fatal catatonia, acute delirious mania, manic-depressive exhaustion death, psychotic exhaustion syndrome, hypertoxic schizophrenia, delirium acutum, delire aigu, and Scheid's cyanotic syndrome* (Mann et al. 1986). Perhaps the most frequently cited article was written by Stauder (1934), who coined the term *lethal catatonia*; for many years, this term was the most widely used designation for this condition. More recently, Philbrick and Rummans (1994), stressing that not all cases prove fatal, have promulgated the term *malignant catatonia* (MC), which we use here as a generic term for this disorder.

MC has remained widely discussed in reports from Europe and Asia. In contrast, North American publications on MC over the past 50 years have been more limited, with an almost complete lack of reference to the current foreign work or reports from the pre–antipsychotic drug era. In this chapter, we provide a comprehensive review of the historical and modern world literature on MC. On the basis of this review, we believe that MC continues to occur and represents an uncommon but potentially lethal neuropsychiatric disorder characterized by severe hyperthermia. Despite the likely decline in its prevalence worldwide, coincident with the introduction of modern psychopharmacological agents, lack of recognition probably accounts for the scarcity of more recent North American reports on MC. Furthermore, our review indicates that MC is a syndrome rather than a specific disease. Although most often presenting as an outgrowth of the major psychoses, MC also may occur in association with diverse neuromedical conditions. In this way, MC resembles "simple, nonmalignant catatonia," which is also a nonspecific response of the central nervous system associated with various neurological, toxic-metabolic, infectious, and psychiatric conditions.

Substantial controversy surrounds the relation between simple catatonia, MC, and neuroleptic malignant syndrome (NMS). Although some consider these conditions to be separate diagnostic entities (Castillo et al. 1989; Fleischhacker et al. 1990), others conclude that they are part of a unitary syndrome (Fink 1996; Fricchione et al. 1997; Tignol and Meggle 1989; D.A.C. White and Robins 2000). In this chapter, we draw on data from our review to address this controversy and provide evidence that NMS represents an iatrogenic, antipsychotic drug–induced form of MC. Furthermore, we suggest that catatonia, MC, and NMS share a common pathophysiology involving reduced dopaminergic neurotransmission within the basal ganglia–thalamocortical circuits. A view of these disorders as manifestations of a single clinical entity has important implications for timely recognition, differential diagnosis, and treatment.

🔖 Clinical Presentation: Pre–Antipsychotic Drug Era

Alzheimer, Kraepelin, and Bleuler were among the many physicians of the pre–antipsychotic drug era to discuss MC (Mann et al. 1986). Despite the remarkable diversity of nomenclature, early clinical accounts of MC had considerable consistency and suggested the following composite clinical

---

TABLE 5–1.   Clinical features of malignant catatonia

Prodromal phase
   Average duration: 2 weeks
Hyperactive phase
   Average duration: 8 days (1 day to several weeks)
      Extreme motoric excitement
      Refusal of all foods and fluids
      Clouding of consciousness
      Somatic disturbances
      Catatonic signs
      Hyperthermia
Final stage
   Duration: <4 days
   Stuporous exhaustion (musculature flaccid or rigid, coma, cardiovascular
      collapse, and death)

---

sketch (Table 5–1). A prodromal phase lasting an average of 2 weeks, but ranging from a few days to several months, was noted in most, but not all, cases. This phase was characterized by lability of mood, with various degrees of depression, anxiety, perplexity, and euphoria. Sleep deteriorated markedly, and delusions and hallucinations often appeared. Stauder (1934) stated that such prodromal signs "cannot be distinguished from the beginnings of other schizophrenias" (p. 623). In about 90% of the cases reported during the pre–antipsychotic drug era, the disease proper began with a phase of extreme motoric excitement, which then continued night and day almost without interruption. Shulack's (1946) account is representative. He described excitement, which progressed to

> A continual maniacal furor, in which the individual will tear off his clothes, tear the clothes to strips, take the bed apart, rip the mattress to pieces, bang and pound almost rhythmically on the walls and windows, dash wildly from the room, assault anyone in reach and run aimlessly and without objective.... If placed in restraints, he will strain ceaselessly. (p. 466)

At times, excitement might be interrupted by periods of catatonic stupor and rigidity. Other catatonic signs such as mutism, catalepsy, staring, posturing, echolalia, and echopraxia were often noted during this excited phase. Thought processes became increasingly disorganized, and speech grew progressively incoherent. Auditory and visual hallucinations accompanied by bizarre delusions were often prominent. Clouding of consciousness was observed in most cases and was viewed by many investigators as one of the cardinal features of the disorder.

Refusal of all foods and fluids was characteristic of the excited phase, leading to cachexia and dehydration. The pulse became rapid, even in periods of momentary rest. Blood pressure was labile, the skin was pale, and perspiration was profuse. Acrocyanosis and spontaneous hematomas of the skin were frequently noted. In this "classic" excited form of MC, excitement was always associated with hyperthermia, which often attained levels above 43.3°C prior to the final stuporous phase of the disorder. This differs phenomenologically from NMS in that although NMS is often preceded by a period of hyperactivity, hyperthermia first emerges concomitantly with, or shortly after, the onset of stupor and rigidity. The excited phase of MC varied in duration from less than a day to several weeks but lasted an average of 8 days (Arnold and Stepan 1952).

In the final phase of the disorder, excitement gave way to stuporous exhaustion, with extreme hyperthermia followed by coma, cardiovascular collapse, and death. In many reports, skeletal musculature was described as rigid during this terminal stupor, similar to that seen in NMS. Stauder (1934), for instance, observed that after the peak of psychomotor excitement, all 27 patients in his series passed through a stage during which they became extremely rigid and would "lay [*sic*] in bed with clenched teeth, each muscle tensed" (p. 627) and would exhibit bizarre posturing. In Stauder's (1934) series, terminal rigidity and stupor lasted 36 hours to 4 days. Conversely, other reports noted musculature to be flaccid (Arnold and Stepan 1952). This differs from NMS, in which muscular rigidity is a cardinal feature. It must be emphasized that about 10% of the cases reported during the pre–antipsychotic drug era involved catatonic stupor and hyperthermia unassociated with a preceding excited phase—that is, they had a primarily stuporous course.

Laboratory abnormalities included increases in erythrocyte sedimentation rate, blood urea nitrogen, and serum potassium and chloride and decreased serum calcium. Leukocytosis and lymphopenia were sometimes present. A variety of coagulation abnormalities were variably described. Stauder (1934) and Arnold and Stepan (1952) reported findings consistent with a familial occurrence of MC. During most of the pre–antipsychotic drug era, MC was reported fatal in 75% (Bell 1849) to 100% (Lingjaerde 1963) of cases. Most reports were in agreement with Scheideggar's (1929) observations that MC occurred predominantly in young adults between ages 18 and 35 and involved women about seven times more often than men. During this early period, MC was estimated to account for 0.25% (Ladame 1919) to 3.5% (Derby 1933) of admissions to psychiatric hospitals. MC was reported to occur with equal frequency throughout the seasons, similar to NMS. Of particular interest was a report by Derby (1933) discussing 187 "manic-depressive exhaustion deaths"; hyperactive manic patients would seem particularly vulnerable to summer heat. However, this report also indicated a uniform seasonal distribution.

Most early French researchers viewed MC as a specific disease rather than a nonspecific syndrome (Ladame 1919). Certain inflammatory and degenerative changes found on autopsy, although often quite mild, were nevertheless considered clear evidence of a rare but deadly form of encephalitis preferentially involving the hypothalamus. In contrast, Kraepelin (1905) and Scheideggar (1929) were among a number of German researchers of this period who considered MC a clinical syndrome, composed of characteristic symptoms and a set course but lacking a specific etiology. They believed that MC could occur as an outgrowth of various neuromedical illnesses as well as in association with the major psychoses. Huber (1954) stated that aside from occurring within the context of schizophrenia, MC could develop as a complication of general paresis, brain tumors, cerebrovascular accidents, brain trauma (especially trauma involving the frontal lobes), seizure disorders, various intoxications, and infectious disorders. In addition, Huber (1954) mentioned cases of MC "superimposed on unclassifiable brain processes" that presented as an "atypical encephalitis" involving lymphocytic and plasmacytic perivascular infiltrates not unlike the findings described by previous French researchers (Ladame 1919).

Subsequent to Stauder's (1934) publication, however, MC was increasingly viewed as confined to the major psychoses, although Stauder himself never fully dismissed the possibility that some or all of his patients may have had encephalitis. Most German investigators came to view MC as an outgrowth of schizophrenia. Jahn and Greving (1936) and Knoll (1954) believed that they were able to identify schizophrenia in most of their patients who developed MC. Arnold and Stepan (1952) followed up 16 survivors of MC for 3 years and found evidence of schizophrenia in 10 (62.5%). However, the remaining 6 patients were symptom free at follow-up.

The opinion of American investigators of this period was more divergent. Billig and Freeman (1944) echoed the German literature, which suggested a decisive link between MC and schizophrenia. In keeping with the line of thought developed by Bell (1849), however, others thought that MC was primarily an outgrowth of mania (Kraines 1934). Although Derby (1933) reported on hyperthermic exhaustion deaths in manic-depressive psychosis, he noted that a similar picture could occur in association with schizophrenia. Shulack (1946) believed that MC could occur with manic-depressive illness, schizophrenia, and postpartum and involutional psychoses.

Most German and American researchers of the pre–antipsychotic drug era emphasized lack of autopsy findings that could account for the cause of death in MC. Any central nervous system abnormalities considered pathognomonic by the French were either unconfirmed or deemed trivial. Post-mortem findings were seen as limited to general visceral and encephalic vascular congestion, with some researchers noting fibrosis in organs outside the central nervous system. Histopathological examination generally found nothing more than mild nonspecific degenerative changes, petechiae, and small hemorrhages in the cerebral cortex and other body organs. Bronchopneumonia or other infections found on autopsy were considered "opportunistic" because they occurred in an already exhausted and compromised host. Such infections were "capable of accelerating death but not representing the sole cause of lethal outcome" (Stauder 1934, p. 628). Kraines (1934) summarized the controversy surrounding autopsy findings by quoting Bell (1849): "Slight cerebral and meningeal engorgements which constituted the only marks of the disease were no greater than the incidents of sleeplessness, agitation, and death might be expected to leave independent of any great morbid action behind these" (Kraines 1934, p. 38).

Prior to the mid-1940s, the mortality of MC continued to exceed 75%. In 1952, Arnold and Stepan reported on the treatment of MC with "shock blocks" of electroconvulsive therapy (ECT). In one study, 16 (84.2%) of 19 patients receiving "shock blocks" within the first 5 days after the onset of MC survived. However, Arnold and Stepan (1952) stressed that early identification of MC and prompt initiation of treatment were critical; none of the 14 patients starting ECT more than 5 days beyond the onset of MC survived. Treatment began with a "block" of three bilateral ECT treatments spaced at 15-minute intervals. The fourth ECT treatment was given 8–24 hours later, depending on the clinical condition. Following this, one to two treatments were given daily for the next 2–3 days, followed by treatments on alternate days or twice weekly to a total of 12–15 treatments.

🗐 Contemporary Literature

Since the mid-1980s, we have reviewed the world literature on several occasions to assess the current status of MC (Lazarus et al. 1989; Mann and Caroff 1990; Mann et al. 1986, 1990, 2001, 2002, in press). In our first article (Mann et al. 1986), we identified a series of 292 cases reported between 1960 and 1985. Two hundred sixty-five cases came from 20 reports representative of more than 50 publications from Europe and Asia. The remaining 27 cases were reported in 12 articles found in an exhaustive search of the post-1960 North American literature. Fifteen of these 27 cases came from a single study that provided little specific detail. Most patients had received antipsychotics. Since then, we have identified 77 additional MC cases reported in the world literature between 1986 and 2002, thus extending our series to 369 contemporary cases. Of note, 25 of the most recent 77 MC cases were found in 18 North American reports, and the remaining 52 came from 35 European and Asian publications. Although MC remains more frequently mentioned in the foreign literature, the disparity now appears reduced, suggesting improved recognition of this disorder in North America.

In 322 cases in which sex was specified, 212 (65.8%) were female. This indicates that women continue to be more commonly affected, although the trend may now be somewhat reduced. The mean age at occurrence was 33, compared with 25 during the pre–antipsychotic drug era. Patient age ranged from 13 to 79 years, contrasting with the belief of some early investigators that MC occurs primarily in the second and third decades of life. Of the 369 patients, 183 (50.0%) died, representing a modest reduction from the pre–antipsychotic drug era when mortality ranged from 75% to 100%. However, among the 77 cases reported since 1986, only 7 (9.1%) ended in death. This apparent decline in mortality is striking and presumably reflects greater awareness of MC, early diagnosis, and the rapid institution of appropriate management strategies. Nevertheless, MC continues to represent a potentially lethal disorder. Similar to findings from the pre–antipsychotic drug era, a uniform seasonal distribution was evident. Among cases reported since 1960, MC was estimated to occur in 0.07% of psychiatric admissions (Koziel-Schminda 1973) or annually in 0.0004% of community adults (Hafner and Kasper 1982). Aside from catatonic hyperactivity and stupor, the clinical features of MC described in this literature are hyperthermia, altered consciousness, and autonomic instability as manifested by diaphoresis, tachycardia, labile or elevated blood pressure, and varying degrees of cyanosis. Catatonic signs aside from stupor and excitement continue to be noted. In one large series from our review, Singerman and Raheja (1994) identified 62 patients with psychogenic MC and reported that each had more than two catatonic features. Among our 77 most recent MC cases, muscular rigidity was reported in 27 (79.4%) of 34 patients in whom muscle tone was characterized.

In our original series of 292 cases (Mann et al. 1986), creatine phosphokinase (CPK) levels had been obtained in only three patients and were elevated in two. Among the 77 recent MC cases, CPK was elevated in 24 (96.0%) of 25 patients in whom it was tested. In this most recent series, leukocytosis was reported in 17 (70.8%) of 24 patients, and hepatic transaminases were elevated in 10 (50%) of 20 patients. Serum iron levels were obtained in only seven patients but were decreased in all seven. Less consistent findings among the 77 recent cases included nonfocal generalized slowing on electroencephalography, mild hyperglycemia, elevated serum creatinine, hyponatremia, hypernatremia, and dehydration. Philbrick and

Rummans (1994) found that three of five patients with MC treated at their facility had evidence of frontal atrophy on computed tomography (CT) scans of the head. Furthermore, one patient with a normal head CT scan had decreased frontal perfusion on posttreatment single photon emission computed tomography. Among the recent 77 cases, neuroimaging findings consistent with frontal atrophy were noted in three additional patients with psychogenic MC.

Forty-nine (13.3%) of the full sample of 369 contemporary MC cases were believed to be caused by diverse neuromedical conditions. Reports of infectious causes included 19 cases of acute or postinfectious viral encephalitis (Abczynska and Terminska 1995; Dekleva and Husain 1995; Johnson and Lucey 1987; Mann et al. 1986; Prabhakar et al. 1992; Rubin 1978; Shill and Stacey 2000; Volkow et al. 1987); single cases of *Borrelia* encephalitis (Neumarker et al. 1989), general paresis (Mann et al. 1986), bacterial meningoencephalitis (Orland and Daghestani 1987), viral hepatitis (Mann et al. 1986), and bacterial septicemia that evolved from five cases of endometritis (Mann et al. 1986); and single cases each of pyelonephritis, tuberculosis of the large intestine, aortitis, cholangitis, endocarditis, and gingival abscess (Mann et al. 1986). In two patients who developed MC of septic origin, the original focus of infection was not indicated (Mann et al. 1986). Cerebrovascular thrombosis accounted for two cases (Mann et al. 1986), whereas MC developed in the context of normal-pressure hydrocephalus in another (Philbrick and Rummans 1994). Reports of metabolic disorders causing MC included two cases of hyperthyroidism (Mann et al. 1986) and single cases of uremia (Mann et al. 1986), systemic lupus erythematosus (Fricchione et al. 1990), and cerebral anoxia (Mann et al. 1986). Reports of toxic causes of MC included single cases due to tetraethyl lead poisoning, sedative-hypnotic withdrawal, renal transplantation (Mann et al. 1986), toxic epidermal necrolysis (Weller and Kornhuber 1992a, 1992b), and therapeutic ingestion or overdose of cyclobenzaprine (Theoharides et al. 1995).

Of the 369 cases, 320 (86.7%) were considered the outgrowth of a major psychotic disorder, diagnosed as schizophrenia in 126 cases, mania in 13 cases, major depression in 22 cases, psychosis not otherwise specified in 22 cases, and "periodic catatonia" in 10 cases. In the remaining 127 cases of psychogenic origin, a specific diagnosis was not given. In this series, the frequent association of MC with schizophrenia may be spurious, resulting from a continued misconception that catatonic signs imply catatonic schizophrenia. Because considerable evidence suggests that simple psychogenic catatonia may more commonly represent the expression of a mood disorder (M.A. Taylor 1990), the frequency with which MC develops in association with mood disorders may not yet be adequately appreciated. Of the 320 MC cases attributed to the major psychoses, 163 (50.9%) cases ended in death. Autopsy data were available for 99. Of these 99 cases, 79 (79.8%) proved autopsy negative and, as such, were considered "genuine" psychogenic MC cases. In the remaining 20 cases, however, death could be attributed to specific consequences of catatonic immobility, such as deep venous thrombosis with pulmonary embolism. Such cases of simple psychogenic catatonia rendered fatal by severe intercurrent medical complications were differentiated from genuine psychogenic MC.

🖋 Catatonia, Malignant Catatonia, and Neuroleptic Malignant Syndrome

Our review of the modern world literature on MC supports Kraepelin's (1905) belief that MC represents a syndrome rather than a specific disease and that it may occur in association with diverse neuromedical disorders as well as with the major psychoses. In addition to the neuromedical causes of MC identified in our review, clinical pictures like that of MC, although not identified as such, are found elsewhere in the medical literature. Table 5–2 summarizes known causes of the MC syndrome.

Consistent with a conceptualization of MC as a nonspecific syndrome, it is appropriate to consider its relation to simple catatonia and NMS. Among the 369 contemporary MC cases, the "classic" excited form involving extreme hyperactivity and progressive hyperthermia prior to the onset of stupor continued to predominate, with 67% of cases presenting in this fashion. However, 33% of the patients had a primarily stuporous course. This represents a change from the pre–antipsychotic drug era, when only about 10% of patients presented in this fashion. Furthermore, a selective analysis of the 77 MC cases reported since 1986 indicated that this trend has continued, with 57% showing excitement and 43% now presenting as stuporous. In many of these cases involving a primarily stuporous course, stupor and hyperthermia developed only following the initiation of antipsychotic drug treatment, giving rise to questions about the demarcation of MC from NMS. Furthermore, the clinical features of "classic" excited MC, once stupor emerges, appear equally difficult to distinguish from NMS. Viewing MC as a syndrome that may occur as an outgrowth of both the major psychoses and diverse neuromedical conditions, we have suggested that NMS represents an antipsychotic drug–induced toxic or iatrogenic form of MC.

Along these lines, Rummans and associates (Philbrick and Rummans 1994; Rummans 2000) viewed catatonia as a spectrum with milder forms at one end (termed *simple* or *nonmalignant*) and more severe forms, involving

TABLE 5–2.   Disorders associated with malignant catatonia syndrome

Psychiatric disorders
    Schizophrenia
    Mood disorders
    Periodic catatonia
    Psychotic disorder not otherwise specified

Cerebrovascular disorders
    Basilar artery thrombosis
    Bilateral hemorrhagic infarction of the anterior cingulate gyri
    Bilateral hemorrhagic lesions of the temporal lobes

Other central nervous system causes
    Normal-pressure hydrocephalus
    Seizure disorders
        Autonomic (diencephalic) epilepsy
        Petit mal status
    Cerebral anoxia

Tumors
    Periventricular diffuse pinealoma
    Glioma of the third ventricle
    Glioma involving the splenum of the corpus callosum
    Angioma of the midbrain

Head trauma
    Closed head trauma
    Surgical removal of lesions near the hypothalamus

Infections
    Viral encephalitis—acute or postinfectious
    Borrelia encephalitis
    Bacterial meningoencephalitis
    General paresis
    Viral hepatitis
    Bacterial septicemia

Metabolic disorders
    Hyperthyroidism
    Addison's disease
    Cushing's disease
    Uremia
    Wernicke's encephalopathy
    Systemic lupus erythematosus

Toxic disorders
    Postoperative states
    Sedative-hypnotic withdrawal
    Tetraethyl lead poisoning
    Cyclobenzaprine toxicity
    Toxic epidermal necrolysis
    Neuroleptic malignant syndrome

Source.   Adapted from Mann SC, Caroff SN, Bleier HR, et al.: "Lethal Catatonia." *American Journal of Psychiatry* 143:1374–1381, 1986. Used with permission. Copyright 1986 American Psychiatric Association.

hyperthermia and autonomic dysfunction (termed *malignant*), at the other. Stressing that catatonia has both neuromedical and psychiatric etiologies, they too conceptualized NMS as an antipsychotic drug–induced form of MC and thus another variant of the larger catatonic syndrome. Similarly, noting that antipsychotics are a well-known cause of catatonia, Fricchione (1985; Fricchione et al. 1997, 2000) suggested a close relation between catatonic states triggered by antipsychotics and those that are not and proposed that antipsychotic drug–induced catatonia is to simple catatonia as NMS is to MC. Goforth and Carroll (1995) provided further evidence for overlap between the diagnoses of catatonia and NMS. Among 27 cases of NMS, all met the DSM-IV (American Psychiatric Association 1994) diagnostic criteria for catatonia, whereas 24 met much stricter research criteria. The authors concluded that the two syndromes are identical, with NMS presenting as a severe iatrogenic variant of MC. Recently, these findings were replicated by Koch et al. (2000), who reported that 15 (93.8%) of 16 patients with NMS met simultaneous clinical and research criteria for catatonia. Furthermore, in each of their cases, Koch et al. (2000) reported a strong positive correlation between the severity of NMS and the number of catatonic signs recorded, strengthening the argument for a relation between the two disorders and consistent with a view of NMS as a severe variant of catatonia. Fink (1996, 2001) also contended that NMS and catatonia are variants of the same disorder.

In 1991, Rosebush and Mazurek found decreased serum iron levels in NMS and suggested a role for lowered iron stores in impairing dopamine receptor function in that disorder. In support of the hypothesis that NMS is a severe variant of catatonia, Carroll and Goforth (1995) reported a similar decrease in serum iron in 3 of 12 catatonic episodes, with NMS developing in 2 of the 3 episodes. The third episode did not involve antipsychotic drug exposure and did not progress to NMS. J.W.Y. Lee (1998) prospectively identified 50 patients with catatonia; serum iron levels were measured in 39 catatonic episodes. A low serum iron level was reported in 17 (43.6%) episodes and was associated with MC and a poor response to benzodiazepines. Serum iron levels were low in all 7 MC episodes identified in this series. Of note, J.W.Y. Lee (1998) distinguished MC from NMS based on an absence of "extrapyramidal features" in this study. He reported that when antipsychotic drug treatment was initiated in 5 MC episodes, all progressed to NMS.

D.A.C. White and Robins (1991, 2000) reported important clinical observations indicating that patients with catatonia may be at increased risk for developing NMS. In 1991, D.A.C. White and Robins described five consecutive cases of NMS in which catatonia had been the presenting picture before the administration of antipsychotic drugs. Since then, these

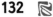

investigators have reported a similar sequence of prodromal catatonia leading to NMS in 12 more consecutive cases. In 9 cases, catatonia progressed
to NMS after a single antipsychotic dose. Of particular interest was one patient from the series (D.A.C. White 1992) who had multiple separate episodes of MC and NMS. In this case, the only clinical feature that appeared
to differentiate MC from NMS episodes was the presence of muscular rigidity in NMS. On the basis of the above observations, the investigators argued that NMS represents an intensification of a preexisting catatonic state
and is not a separate diagnostic entity.

In contrast, some investigators consider simple catatonia, MC, and
NMS to be distinct clinical syndromes (Castillo et al. 1989; Fleischhacker
et al. 1990; J.W.Y. Lee and Robertson 1997; Theoharides et al. 1995).
Both Castillo et al. (1989) and Fleischhacker et al. (1990) proposed that excited or agitated behavior points to a diagnosis of MC. However, agitation
is a common feature of the psychosis preceding NMS for which antipsychotics were originally used (Ahuja and Nehru 1990; Levenson 1989).
Castillo et al. (1989) maintained that prominent muscular rigidity might be
a distinguishing feature. Similarly, J.W.Y. Lee (1998) differentiated NMS
from "non-NMS MC" on the basis of extrapyramidal rigidity. However, as
Levenson (1989) underscored, patients with agitated catatonia usually receive antipsychotics early in treatment. As such, if rigidity is present, it may
be difficult to know whether this represents NMS or antipsychotic drug–
induced extrapyramidal symptoms superimposed on MC. Furthermore, in
our most recent series of 77 MC cases, muscular rigidity was identified in
79% of the cases in which its presence or absence was specified.

Other investigators have argued that case reports and case series studies of NMS do not consistently mention catatonic features (J.W.Y. Lee
1998, 2000; Lohr and Wisenewski 1987). J.W.Y. Lee (2000) proposed that
NMS be viewed as a heterogeneous condition with "catatonic" and "non-
catatonic NMS" representing two major subgroups. Previously, Caroff et
al. (1998a) asserted that catatonia in NMS appears primarily as mutism and
akinesia, whereas the verbal, bizarre, and hyperkinetic signs that can be
elicited in some catatonic patients are infrequently reported. Pearlman
(2000) reviewed approximately 700 reports of NMS contained in the world
literature between 1989 and 1999 and found that catatonic features were
mentioned in only 25% of the cases. However, Pearlman (2000) underscored that incomplete reporting of clinical data in these cases compromised attempts to assess the actual prevalence of catatonic features. This
contrasts with the work of Goforth and Carroll (1995), Koch et al. (2000),
and Francis and Petrides (1998), in which NMS patients were systematically screened for catatonia with specific catatonia rating scales.

Of considerable interest, Carroll and Taylor (1997) conducted a retrospective review of patients with chart diagnoses of either MC or NMS and attempted to differentiate them with the criteria proposed by Castillo et al. (1989). They compared 9 cases of NMS with 17 MC cases but could find no predominance of either MC or NMS features as outlined by Castillo et al. (1989). Thus, the clinical phenomenology failed to distinguish the two syndromes in this retrospective comparison. Based on our review of the literature, we concur with Fricchione and colleagues' (1997, 2000) conclusion that despite a few subtle differences in presentation, MC and NMS appear to be part of a unitary catatonic syndrome. Accordingly, the emergence of NMS as an antipsychotic drug–induced subtype of MC could help explain the increased percentage of MC cases involving a primarily stuporous course reported in the contemporary world literature.

Pathogenesis

A consideration of the pathogenesis of MC with a particular focus on dopamine further supports a view of simple catatonia, MC, and NMS as variants of a unitary syndrome. Numerous investigators have posited a key role for central dopaminergic hypoactivity in triggering both simple catatonia and MC (Fricchione 1985; Fricchione et al. 1997, 2000; Lohr and Wisenewski 1987; Philbrick and Rummans 1994; M.A. Taylor 1990). Furthermore, compelling clinical evidence implicates antipsychotic drug–induced dopamine receptor blockade in the pathogenesis of NMS (Mann et al. 1991, 2000). Recently, Fricchione et al. (1997, 2000) along with our group (Mann et al. 2000, 2002) proposed that the onset of catatonia coincides with a reduction in dopaminergic activity within the basal ganglia–thalamocortical circuits. Alexander (1994; Alexander et al. 1986, 1990) characterized these frontal-subcortical circuits as one of the brain's principal organizational networks underlying brain-behavior relationships. Five circuits connecting the basal ganglia with their associated areas in the cortex and thalamus have been identified and are named according to their function or cortical site of origin (Figure 5–1). They include the "motor circuit," the "oculomotor circuit," the "dorsolateral prefrontal circuit," the "lateral orbitofrontal circuit," and the "anterior cingulate–medial orbitofrontal circuit." Each circuit involves the same member structures, including an origin in a specific area of the frontal cortex; projections to the striatum (putamen, caudate, and ventral striatum); connections to the globus pallidus interna (GPi) and the substantia nigra pars reticulata (SNr), which, in turn, project to specific thalamic nuclei; and a final link back to the frontal area from which they originated, thus creating a feedback loop (Figure 5–1).

In addition, within each circuit are dual opposing pathways linking the

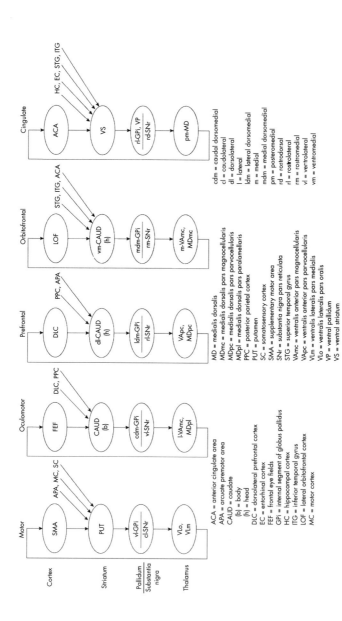

FIGURE 5–1. Proposed basal ganglia–thalamocortical circuits.

Parallel organization of the five basal ganglia–thalamocortical circuits. Each circuit engages specific regions of the cerebral cortex, striatum, pallidum, substantia nigra, and thalamus.

Source. Adapted from Alexander et al. 1986.

striatum with the Gpi and SNr that represent the major outflow nuclei of the basal ganglia circuitry (Figure 5–2): a *direct* monosynaptic pathway from the striatum to the Gpi and SNr and an *indirect* pathway from the striatum to the globus pallidus externa (Gpe) and then to the subthalamic nucleus (STN) before connecting with the Gpi and SNr. Each of the five circuits uses the same neurotransmitters in relaying information between analogous anatomical sites (Cummings 1993). Dopamine is in a key position to influence activity in each of the circuits (Lou 1998; Mega and Cummings 1994; Mega et al. 1997). Mesocortical dopaminergic pathways project directly to circuit origin sites in the supplementary motor area, frontal eye fields, and the three prefrontal cortical areas. Additionally, dopamine modulates each circuit through its projections to the striatum (Cummings 1993). Although significant overlap exists, most dopaminergic input to the dorsal striatum (caudate and putamen) comes from the substantia nigra pars compacta (SNc) (nigrostriatal pathway), whereas the ventral tegmentum provides the bulk of dopaminergic innervation to the ventral striatum (mesolimbic pathway). Furthermore, within the circuits, dopamine has differential effects on the direct and the indirect pathways. The motor, the anterior cingulate–medial orbitofrontal, and the lateral orbitofrontal circuits represent major candidates for involvement in the pathogenesis of simple catatonia, MC, and NMS.

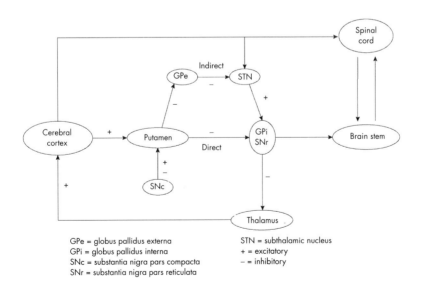

GPe = globus pallidus externa
GPi = globus pallidus interna
SNc = substantia nigra pars compacta
SNr = substantia nigra pars reticulata

STN = subthalamic nucleus
+ = excitatory
– = inhibitory

FIGURE 5–2. Basal ganglia–thalamocortical "motor" circuit.
Source. Reprinted from Lou J-S: "Pathophysiology of Basal Ganglia Disorders." *CNS Spectrums* 3:36–40, 1998. Used with permission.

Hypodopaminergia involving the motor circuit could account for muscular rigidity and contribute to akinesia in these conditions (Mann et al. 2000) (Figure 5–2). The motor circuit originates from neurons in the supplementary motor area and parts of the motor, premotor, and somatosensory areas that project topographically to the putamen (Figure 5–1). This projection, like all circuit pathways between the cortex and the striatum, is glutamatergic and hence excitatory (Alexander 1994). The putamen then projects both a direct and an indirect pathway to the GPi and SNr (Figure 5–2). The direct pathway uses γ-aminobutyric acid (GABA) as its transmitter and is inhibitory. Cortical activation of the direct pathway thus produces a suppression of GPi and SNr output, which is itself GABA-ergic and inhibitory, thereby disinhibiting the thalamus. The thalamus is then free to send excitatory glutamatergic projections to the circuit's cortical area of origin. The net effect is that the direct pathway provides positive feedback for cortically initiated movements and has a principal role in sustaining ongoing patterns of motor behavior. In contrast, cortical activation of the indirect pathway inhibits the GPe, which uses GABA to disinhibit the STN (Lou 1998). The excitatory STN sends a glutamatergic projection that drives the GPi and SNr to inhibit the thalamus. This then suppresses excitatory thalamic feedback to the cortex. The net effect is that the indirect pathway provides negative feedback for cortically initiated movements and is used to suppress ongoing patterns of motor behavior (Alexander 1994).

Consistent with the basal ganglia–thalamocortical circuit organization, dopamine exerts differential effects on the direct and indirect pathways. Nigrostriatal dopaminergic input excites GABA-ergic putaminal neurons projecting to the GPi and SNr via the direct pathway but inhibits those projecting to the GPe via the indirect pathway (Lou 1998) (Figure 5–2). As such, a reduction in dopaminergic functioning associated with the onset of the catatonic syndrome would suppress activity in the direct pathway, where dopamine facilitates transmission, but enhance activity in the indirect pathway, where dopamine is inhibitory. The overall outcome would be increased output from the GPi and SNr yielding excessive inhibition of thalamocortical neurons, as is believed to occur in Parkinson's disease (Lou 1998). In particular, increased activity in the indirect pathway, which is used to suppress motor activity, could cause muscular rigidity and contribute to akinesia in simple catatonia, MC, and NMS.

The anterior cingulate–medial orbitofrontal subcortical circuit may mediate diminished arousal, mutism, and akinesia in simple catatonia, MC, and NMS and also may participate in causing hyperthermia and autonomic dysfunction (Mann et al. 2000). This circuit engages some cortical and subcortical structures that are thought to be limbic in nature (Alexander et al.

1990). It originates in the anterior cingulate area, the medial orbitofrontal area, and the association cortex of the temporal lobe (Figure 5–1). These areas then project to the ventral striatum or *limbic striatum*, which is composed of the nucleus accumbens, the ventromedial part of the caudate putamen, and the olfactory tubercle. The ventral striatum provides input to the ventral pallidum, the rostromedial GPi, and the rostrodorsal SNr (Figure 5–1). In addition, the ventral striatum may project an indirect pathway through the medial STN to the ventral pallidum (Mega and Cummings 1994). The ventral pallidum then provides input to the dorsal nucleus of the thalamus, which projects back to the anterior cingulate and medial orbitofrontal areas, completing the circuit. Furthermore, it is of considerable interest that projections from the ventral pallidum to the medial STN extend to the medial aspect of the entopeduncular nucleus of the lateral hypothalamus (Deutch et al. 1993). This suggests that reduced dopaminergic activity could cause hyperthermia and autonomic dysfunction in MC and NMS by disrupting anterior cingulate–medial orbitofrontal transmission to the lateral hypothalamus.

In the first edition of this book, we had suggested that the neurological condition akinetic mutism could serve as a model for mutism, diminished arousal, and akinesia in catatonic states. Akinetic mutism, which involves severe hypomotility, diminished arousal, and mutism, has been mistaken for simple psychogenic catatonia (Mann et al. 1991, 2000). Furthermore, certain cases of this disorder have involved hyperthermia and autonomic dysfunction, making them difficult to distinguish from MC and NMS. Akinetic mutism has resulted from various bilateral lesions of the centromedial brain, including brain stem areas, periventricular nuclei of the hypothalamus, the mammillary bodies, and the anterior cingulate area. This distribution of lesions is highly correlated with the anatomical location of the mesocortical dopamine pathway to the anterior cingulate area as it courses rostrally in the medial forebrain bundle. Accordingly, this appeared to support a pathogenetic role for reduced dopaminergic neurotransmission in the mesocortical dopaminergic pathway to the anterior cingulate area in causing mutism, diminished arousal, and akinesia in simple catatonia, MC, and NMS.

However, the identification of the basal ganglia–thalamocortical circuits suggests an important role for the anterior cingulate–medial orbitofrontal circuit in mediating the effects of hypodopaminergia. Thus, decreased dopaminergic transmission from the ventral tegmental area to the ventral striatum would be propagated via the anterior cingulate–medial orbitofrontal circuit to the ventral pallidum, and then to the anterior thalamic nucleus, and ultimately to the anterior cingulate (Figure 5–1), resulting in decreased excitatory input to that area. This latter pathway would appear particularly important for the pathogenesis of antipsychotic drug–induced catatonia and NMS; in these conditions, direct participation of the mesocortical dopaminergic pathway would seem unlikely, in view of the predominance of D_1 and D_4 over D_2 dopamine receptors in the cerebral cortex (Meador-Woodruff et al. 1996).

The lateral orbitofrontal subcortical circuit may account for selected catatonic features observed in simple catatonia, MC, and NMS (Mann et al. 2000). The lateral orbitofrontal circuit originates in the lateral orbitofrontal cortex and projects to the ventromedial sector of the caudate nucleus (Alexander et al. 1990) (Figure 5–1). This part of the caudate projects to the rostromedial SNr and the mediodorsal GPi (Cummings 1993). The rostromedial SNr and the mediodorsal GPi then project to the medial portions of the ventral anterior and medial dorsal thalamic nuclei, which, in turn, project back to the lateral orbitofrontal cortex, closing the circuit. Bilateral lesions of the lateral orbitofrontal cortex or dysfunction in the orbitofrontal circuit have been associated with use and imitation behaviors (Cummings 1993; Mega and Cummings 1994). These behaviors involve automatic imitation of the gestures and actions of others or automatic and inappropriate use of objects such as tools or utensils. As Cummings (1993) pointed out, use and imitation behaviors reflect enslavement to environmental cues. These behaviors share striking similarities with catatonic features such as echopraxia, echolalia, and gegenhalten, all of which are viewed as stimulus-bound or motor perseverative phenomena consistent with frontal lobe dysfunction (M.A. Taylor 1990). Catatonic signs such as mutism, akinesia, and rigidity may better correlate with perturbations in the motor and anterior cingulate–medial orbitofrontal circuits, as considered above. However, it seems reasonable to propose that the lateral orbitofrontal circuit may mediate use and imitation-like catatonic features in simple catatonia, MC, and NMS.

Our review of the anterior cingulate–medial orbitofrontal circuit indicated that hypodopaminergia within its corticolateral hypothalamic circuitry might contribute to hyperthermia and autonomic dysfunction in MC and NMS. However, as detailed in Chapter 2, substantial evidence supports a prominent role for dopamine in hypothalamic central thermoregulatory heat-loss pathways. Accordingly, reduced dopaminergic neurotransmission involving intrinsic hypothalamic dopamine neurons may be paramount in accounting for hyperthermia in MC and NMS. In addition, dopamine neurons of the A11 group located periventricularly in the dorsal hypothalamus, posterior hypothalamus, and caudal thalamus give rise to a diencephalospinal dopaminergic pathway (Mann et al. 1991, 2000). This pathway provides dopaminergic innervation to the intermediolateral spinal column mediating inhibition of preganglionic sympathetic neurons. As such, hypodopaminergia in this pathway could contribute to autonomic dysfunction in these conditions.

In Chapter 1, we proposed that in addition to D_2 dopamine receptor blockade, NMS is the product of preexisting central dopaminergic hypoactivity that represents a trait vulnerability marker for this disorder, coupled with state-related adjustments in the dopamine system occurring in response to exposure to stress. Here, we suggest that such trait- and state-related factors are also critical in causing hypodopaminergia in the basal ganglia–thalamocortical circuits in simple catatonia and MC. In Chapter 1, we presented several lines of evidence indicating that certain individuals might have baseline hypodopaminergia, including reduced cerebrospinal fluid homovanillic acid (HVA) levels in post-NMS patients (Nisijima and Ishiguro 1990, 1995a); reduced striatal HVA levels or lack of elevated HVA-to-dopamine ratios in three patients who had died of fatal hyperthermia from MC or NMS (Kish et al. 1990); lower cerebrospinal fluid HVA levels and more severe baseline parkinsonian symptoms in 11 patients with Parkinson's disease following their recovery from NMS-like episodes (Ueda et al. 1999); and reports of abnormalities in the D_2 dopamine receptor gene in NMS (Ram et al. 1995; Suzuki et al. 2001) (See Chapter 1 for additional lines of evidence.)

Furthermore, we reviewed findings implicating the enhanced responsiveness of the dopamine system to stress as a state-related cofactor predisposing to NMS-like conditions. As first described more than 25 years ago (Thierry et al. 1976), the dopaminergic innervation of the medial prefrontal cortex in the rat is unique in that it is activated by very mild stressors such as limited footshock stress or conditioned fear paradigms. In addition, considerable data indicate a functional interdependence of dopamine systems innervating the medial prefrontal cortex and subcortical dopamine systems; in particular, changes in the medial prefrontal cortex dopamine system appear to have an inverse relationship to dopamine turnover in the dorsal and ventral striatum (Bubser and Schmidt 1994). Consistent with this, Pycock et al. (1980) showed that lesions of the mesocortical dopamine pathway to the medial prefrontal cortex in the rat result in increased indexes of subcortical dopaminergic functioning.

Conversely, increased mesocortical dopaminergic neurotransmission to the medial prefrontal cortex has been associated with decreased subcortical dopaminergic functioning (Louilot et al. 1989). The latter may be of considerable relevance for understanding the pathogenesis of simple catatonia, MC, and NMS. This model suggests that if acute stress activates the stress-sensitive mesocortical dopaminergic pathway to the medial prefrontal cortex, it will have direct feedback effects in both the dorsal and the ventral striatum, rendering those areas hypodopaminergic and predisposing to simple catatonia, MC, and NMS in individuals with preexisting central dopaminergic hypoactivity. The previous discussion is, of course, simplistic, because other neurotransmitters, including serotonin, GABA, and glutamate, appear directly or indirectly involved in the pathogenesis of these disorders.

🗟 Treatment

Effective management of MC depends on early recognition of this disorder. The potential for severe autonomic symptoms and the high rate of medical complications dictate early institution of intensive medical care focusing on fluid replacement, reduction of temperature, and support of cardiac, respiratory, and renal functions. Careful monitoring for complications, particularly aspiration pneumonia, thromboembolism, and renal failure, is essential. Two reports provide some support for the use of typical antipsychotics in treating early signs of MC and hyperthermia lower than 38°C (Mann et al. 1986). Furthermore, Cassidy et al. (2001) recently reported on an MC case responding to high-dose olanzapine. However, the bulk of evidence indicates that the dopamine receptor blocking effects of antipsychotic drugs are likely to aggravate episodes of MC, as in NMS, in which discontinuation of antipsychotic drug treatment significantly correlates with recovery. In our initial review involving 292 MC cases (Mann et al. 1986), 78% of those treated with only an antipsychotic died, compared with an overall mortality rate of 60%. Furthermore, among the 18 cases reviewed by Philbrick and Rummans (1994), only one patient received treatment with an antipsychotic alone, and that patient died. In view of their questionable efficacy and their clear potential to aggravate MC episodes, antipsychotic drugs should be withheld whenever MC is suspected.

Benzodiazepines have proved highly effective in the treatment of simple catatonia, including antipsychotic drug–induced catatonia (Fricchione et al. 1997, 2000). Furthermore, as discussed in Chapter 1, benzodiazepines have been useful in cases of NMS, particularly those involving milder symptomatology. Philbrick and Rummans (1994) observed that the benefits of benzodiazepines in MC appeared less uniform than in simple catatonia but were nonetheless impressive at times. They asserted that even a partial response to benzodiazepines may be beneficial and retard the progression of MC until more definitive treatment can be instituted. Fricchione et al. (1997, 2000) suggested that if simple catatonia proves unresponsive to benzodiazepines after 5 days of treatment, ECT should be considered as a definitive measure. In MC, however, these researchers argued against a 5-day wait and urged that ECT be started if benzodiazepines do not briskly reverse the MC process.

Indeed, since the previously discussed studies of Arnold and Stepan (1952), ECT has been viewed as a safe and effective treatment for MC when it occurs as an outgrowth of a major psychotic disorder (Mann et al. 1986, 1990, 2001). Although controlled data are lacking, case reports and series of cases have described excellent results with its use. Among 50 patients reported in four larger series from our initial review (Mann et al. 1986), 40 (97.6%) of 41 patients who received ECT survived. In contrast, only 5 of 9 patients who received antipsychotics and supportive care recovered. Similarly, in Philbrick and Rummans' (1994) review of 18 MC cases, 11 (84.6%) of 13 who were given ECT survived, compared with only 1 (20%) of 5 patients who did not receive ECT. However, ECT appears to be effective only if it is initiated before severe progression of MC symptoms. Sedivic (1981) stressed that the development of a comatose state or a temperature in excess of 41°C augurs poorly for psychogenic MC responding even to ECT. Arnold and Stepan (1952) found that in 19 patients starting ECT within 5 days of the onset of hyperthermia, 16 (84.2%) survived, whereas in 14 patients who began treatment beyond this point, ECT had no effect in preventing death. Although earlier protocols called for particularly intensive treatment (e.g., Arnold and Stepan's [1952] "shock blocks"), more recent trials with ECT have indicated that it can be successful when given once daily or every other day for a total of 5–15 treatments (usually unilateral) (Mann et al. 1986, 1990, 2001). Frequently, substantial improvement becomes evident after 1–4 treatments.

Other data, also anecdotal, suggest that MC due to a major psychotic disorder can be effectively treated with corticotropin and corticosteroids (Chrisstoffels and Thiel 1970; Lingjaerde 1963). Lingjaerde (1963) reported that although about 25 MC patients under his care between 1920 and 1949 had all died, the advent of potent hormonal agents since then had led to recovery in 22 (95.7%) of 23 subsequent cases. Chrisstoffels and Thiel (1970) discussed four MC patients successfully treated with corticotropin or corticosteroids and suggested that hormonal agents may be safer than ECT in treating MC. However, since severely debilitated MC patients have generally tolerated ECT without incident, and since the utility of hormonal therapy is less well documented, ECT appears to be the preferred treatment. Corticotropin and corticosteroids may be used if ECT proves ineffective.

In addition, a few cases of MC have been successfully treated with artificial hibernation—that is, the pharmacological induction of hypothermia (Fisher and Greiner 1960). However, this procedure uses phenothiazines, which may worsen the clinical picture, and probably should be avoided. Several investigators have suggested that the addition of dantrolene to ECT represents the optimal treatment for MC (Nolen and Zwann 1990;

Rendfort and Wardin 1985; Van de Kelft et al. 1991), and dantrolene alone has been reported effective in several MC cases (Pennati et al. 1991). Additional cases have involved successful treatment with bromocriptine, dantrolene, and ECT (Goeke et al. 1991); bromocriptine and dantrolene (Singerman and Raheja 1994); bromocriptine and benzodiazepines (Tang et al. 1995); and dantrolene and benzodiazepines (Ferro et al. 1991). Finally, Kaufmann and Wyatt (1987) have advocated the use of calcitonin in the treatment of MC.

In MC occurring as an outgrowth of a neuromedical illness, treatment obviously must be directed at the underlying disorder. Nevertheless, anecdotal reports have described ECT as dramatically effective and at times life saving in suppressing the symptoms of severe MC-like states complicating a diversity of neuromedical conditions (Mann et al. 1986). A.N. Roberts (1963) believed that in such cases, the efficacy of ECT was largely independent of the underlying illness, and improvement was likely to be transient if the neuromedical condition persisted. If, however, the underlying disorder either remits spontaneously or is corrected, permanent recovery may be possible.

▤ Conclusion

MC is a life-threatening hyperthermic neuropsychiatric disorder described long before the introduction of antipsychotic drugs. A review of the world literature on MC indicates that although the prevalence of the condition may have declined since the preantipsychotic drug era, it continues to occur and is now reported more frequently in foreign publications. Lack of recognition probably accounts for the relative paucity of contemporary North American reports on MC. Failure to recognize MC has significant clinical implications. Once developed, this disorder assumes an autonomous and potentially fatal course independent of its etiology. Furthermore, recent findings and findings from the pre–antipsychotic drug era indicate that MC represents a syndrome rather than a specific disease entity. Although most often presenting as an outgrowth of the major psychoses, MC also may occur in association with diverse neuromedical conditions.

Considerable controversy has surrounded the relation among simple catatonia, MC, and NMS. Consistent with a conceptualization of MC as a nonspecific syndrome, we have suggested that NMS represents an iatrogenic, antipsychotic drug–induced form of MC and thus another subtype of the larger catatonic syndrome. Furthermore, the hypothesis that simple catatonia, MC, and NMS share a common pathophysiology involving reduced dopaminergic neurotransmission within the basal ganglia–thalamocortical circuits further supports a view of these disorders as manifestations of a single diagnostic entity. ECT appears to be the preferred treatment for MC stemming from a major psychotic disorder and also may be effective in cases occurring as an outgrowth of a neuromedical illness. However, it is imperative in the latter instance to identify and correct the underlying disorder. Antipsychotic drugs should be withheld whenever MC is suspected.

In this book, we have considered diverse human hyperthermic syndromes resembling NMS that have been recently described as complications of treatment with modern psychopharmacological agents. These reactions may overlap clinically with one another and, in some cases, may share common pathophysiological mechanisms. As discussed in Chapter 1, Delay and associates' (1960) use of the term *syndrome malin des neuroleptiques* evolved from their perception of NMS as an antipsychotic-induced subtype of a more general syndrome malin. As such, syndrome malin appears to overlap conceptually with MC; both define a human hyperthermic syndrome classically associated with psychiatric and neuromedical illnesses and, more recently, recognized in association with contemporary psychopharmacological treatment.

References

Abczynska M, Terminska K: [Psychopathological symptoms in atypical viral hemorrhagic tic borne encephalitis]. Psychiatr Pol 29:547–551, 1995

Abrams R, Taylor MA: EEG observations during combined lithium and neuroleptic treatment. Am J Psychiatry 136:336–337, 1979

Abreo K, Shelp WD, Kosseff A, et al: Amoxapine-associated rhabdomyolysis and acute renal failure: case report. J Clin Psychiatry 43:426–427, 1982

Addonizio G: Rapid induction of extrapyramidal side effects with combined use of lithium and neuroleptics. J Clin Psychopharmacol 5:296–298, 1985

Addonizio G, Susman VL, Roth SD: Symptoms of neuroleptic malignant syndrome in 82 consecutive inpatients. Am J Psychiatry 143:1587–1590, 1986

Addonizio G, Susman VL, Roth SD: Neuroleptic malignant syndrome: review and analysis of 115 cases. Biol Psychiatry 22:1004–1020, 1987

Adityanjee, Singh S, Singh G, et al: Spectrum concept of neuroleptic malignant syndrome. Br J Psychiatry 153:107–111, 1988

Adnet PJ, Krivosic-Horber RM: Neuroleptic malignant syndrome and malignant hyperthermia susceptibility (letter). Acta Anaesthesiol Scand 34:605, 1990

Adnet P, Lestavel P, Krivosic-Horber R: Neuroleptic malignant syndrome. Br J Anaesth 85:129–135, 2000

Ahlenius S, Salmi P: Behavioral and biochemical effects of the dopamine D3 receptor-selective ligand, 7-OH-DPAT, in the normal and reserpine-treated rat. Eur J Pharmacol 260:177–181, 1994

Ahuja N, Nehru R: Neuroleptic malignant syndrome: a subtype of lethal catatonia (letter)? Acta Psychiatr Scand 81:398, 1990

Aisen PS, Lawlor BA: Neuroleptic malignant syndrome induced by low-dose haloperidol (letter). Am J Psychiatry 149:844, 1992

Akpaffiong MJ, Ruiz P: Neuroleptic malignant syndrome: a complication of neuroleptics and cocaine abuse. Psychiatr Q 62:299–309, 1991

Alderman CP, Lee PC: Comment: serotonin syndrome associated with combined sertraline-amitriptyline treatment (letter). Ann Pharmacother 30:1499–1500, 1996

Alexander GE: Basal ganglia-thalamocortical circuits: their role in movements. J Clin Neurophysiol 11:358–370, 1994

Alexander GE, DeLong MR, Strick PL: Parallel organization of functionally segregated circuits linking basal ganglia and cortex. Annu Rev Neurosci 9:357–381, 1986

Alexander GE, Crutcher MD, DeLong MD: Basal ganglia-thalamocortical circuits: parallel substrates for motor, oculomotor, "prefrontal" and "limbic" functions. Prog Brain Res 85:119–146, 1990

Allan RN, White HC: Side effects of parenteral long-acting phenothiazines (letter). BMJ 794:221, 1972

American Psychiatric Association: Diagnostic and Statistical Manual of Mental Disorders, 4th Edition. Washington, DC, American Psychiatric Association, 1994

Amsterdam JD: Selective serotonin reuptake inhibitor efficacy in severe and melancholic depression. J Psychopharmacol 12 (suppl B):S99–S111, 1998

Ananth J, Ruskin R: Unusual reaction to lithium. Can Med Assoc J 111:1049–1050, 1974

Anderson RJ, Reed G, Knochel J: Heatstroke. Adv Intern Med 28:115–140, 1983

Anderson SA, Weinschenk K: Peripheral neuropathy as a component of the neuroleptic malignant syndrome. Am J Med 82:169–170, 1987

Ansseau M, Reynolds CF, Kupfer DJ, et al: Central dopaminergic and noradrenergic receptor blockade in a patient with neuroleptic malignant syndrome. J Clin Psychiatry 47:320–321, 1986

Apte SN, Langston JW: Permanent neurological deficits due to lithium toxicity. Ann Neurol 13:453–455, 1983

Armen R, Kanel G, Reynolds T: Phencyclidine-induced malignant hyperthermia causing submassive liver necrosis. Am J Med 77:167–172, 1984

Arnold OH, Stepan H: Untersuchungen zur Frage der akuten todlichen Katotonie. Wiener Zeitschrift fur Nervenheilkunde und Deren Grenzgebiete 4:235–258, 1952

Asnis GM, Asnis D, Dunner DL, et al: Cogwheel rigidity during chronic lithium therapy. Am J Psychiatry 136:1225–1226, 1979

Auzepy PH, Poivet D, Nitenberg G: Insuffisance respiratoire aigue chez deux schizophrenes (role eventuel des neuroleptiques retards) (letter). La Nouvelle Presse Medicale 6:1236, 1977

Ayd F: Toxic somatic and psychopathologic reactions to antidepressant drugs. J Neuropsychiatry 2 (suppl):119–122, 1961

Ayd FJ Jr: Fatal hyperpyrexia during chlorpromazine therapy. Journal of Clinical and Experimental Psychopathology 17:189–192, 1956

Baastrup PC, Hollnagel P, Sorensen R, et al: Adverse reactions in treatment with lithium carbonate and haloperidol. JAMA 236:2645–2646, 1976

Baetz M, Malcolm D: Serotonin syndrome from fluvoxamine and buspirone (letter). Can J Psychiatry 40:428–429, 1995

Bakkert AMO, Behan PO, Prach AT, et al: A syndrome identical to the neuroleptic malignant syndrome induced by LSD and alcohol. British Journal of Addiction 85:149–151, 1990

Baldessarini RJ: Chemotherapy in Psychiatry, 2nd Edition. Cambridge, MA, Harvard University Press, 1985

Ballard PA, Tetrud JW, Langston JW: Permanent human parkinsonism due to 1-methyl-4-phenyl-1,2,3,6-tetrahydropyridine (MPTP): seven cases. Neurology 35:949–956, 1985

Balster RL: The behavioral pharmacology of phencyclidine, in Psychopharmacology: The Third Generation of Progress. Edited by Meltzer HY. New York, Raven, 1987, pp 1573–1578

Bark N: Deaths of psychiatric patients during heat waves. Psychiatr Serv 49:1088–1090, 1998

Bark NM: Heatstroke in psychiatric patients: two cases and a review. J Clin Psychiatry 43:377–380, 1982

Barnes NM, Sharp T: A review of central 5-HT receptors and their function. Neuropharmacology 38:1083–1152, 1999

Barton CH, Sterling ML, Vaziri ND: Phencyclidine intoxication: clinical experience in 27 cases confirmed by urine assay. Ann Emerg Med 10:243–246, 1981

Bastani JB, Troester MM, Bastani AJ: Serotonin syndrome and fluvoxamine: a case study. Nebraska Medical Journal 50:107–109, 1996

Beaumont G: Drug interactions with clomipramine (Anafranil). J Int Med Res 1:480–484, 1973

Becker T, Kornhuber J, Hoffman E, et al: MRI white matter by hyperintensity in neuroleptic malignant syndrome (NMS)—a clue to pathogenesis? J Neural Transm 90:151–159, 1992

Bedford Russell AR, Schwartz RH, Dawling S: Accidental ingestion of 'Ecstasy' (3,4-methylene dioxymethylamphetamine). Arch Dis Child 67:1114–1115, 1992

Beitman BD: Tardive dyskinesia reinduced by lithium carbonate. Am J Psychiatry 135:1229–1230, 1978

Belfer ML, Shader RI: Autonomic effects, in Psychotropic Drug Side Effects: Clinical and Theoretical Perspectives. Edited by Shader RI, DiMascio A. Baltimore, MD, Williams & Wilkins, 1970, pp 116–123

Bell LV: On a form of disease resembling some advanced stages of mania and fever. American Journal of Insanity 6:97–127, 1849

Belton NR, Backus RE, Millichap JG: Serum creatine phosphokinase activity in epilepsy. Neurology 17:1073–1076, 1967

Benazzi F: Serotonin syndrome with mirtazapine-fluoxetine combination (letter). Int J Geriatr Psychiatry 13:495–496, 1998

Berardi D, Amore M, Keck PE Jr, et al: Clinical and pharmacologic risk factors for neuroleptic malignant syndrome: a case-control study. Biol Psychiatry 44:748–754, 1998

Bettinger J: Cocaine intoxication: massive oral overdose. Ann Emerg Med 9:429–430, 1980

Bhatara VS, Magnus RD, Paul KL, et al: Serotonin syndrome induced by venlafaxine and fluoxetine: a case study in polypharmacy and potential pharmacodynamic and pharmacokinetic mechanisms. Ann Pharmacother 32:432–436, 1998

Biederman J, Lerner Y, Belmaker RH: Combination of lithium carbonate and haloperidol in schizoaffective disorder. Arch Gen Psychiatry 36:327–333, 1979

Billig O, Freeman WT: Fatal catatonia. Am J Psychiatry 100:633–638, 1944

Blier P, Bergeron R: The safety of concomitant use of sumatriptan and antidepressant treatments. J Clin Psychopharmacol 15:106–109, 1995

Blier P, deMontigny C, Chaput Y: Modifications of the serotonin system by antidepressant treatments: implications for the therapeutic response in major depression. J Clin Psychopharmacol 7 (suppl):245–355, 1987

Bligh J, Cottle WH, Maskrey M: Influence of ambient temperature on the thermoregulatory responses to 5-hydroxytryptamine, noradrenaline and acetylcholine injections into the lateral cerebral ventricles of sheep, goats and rabbits. J Physiol 212:377–392, 1971

Bloom FE, Baetge G, Deyo S, et al: Chemical and physiological aspects of the actions of lithium and antidepressant drugs. Neuropharmacology 22:359–365, 1983

Boulant JA: Cellular and synaptic mechanisms of thermosensitivity in hypothalamic neurons, in Thermal Balance in Health and Disease. Edited by Zeisberger E, Schonbaum E, Lomax P. Basel, Switzerland, Birkhauser Verlag AG, 1994, pp 19–29

Boulant JA: Hypothalamic neurons regulating body temperature, in Environmental Physiology: A Critical, Comprehensive Presentation of Physiological Knowledge and Concepts. Edited by Fregly MJ, Blatteis CM. New York, Oxford University Press, 1996, pp 105–126

Boulant JA, Chow AR, Griffin JD: Determinants of hypothalamic neuronal thermosensitivity. Ann N Y Acad Sci 813:133–138, 1997

Boulay D, Depoortere R, Rostene W, et al: Dopamine D-3 receptor agonists produce similar decreases in body temperature and locomotor activity in D-3 knock-out and wild-type mice. Neuropharmacology 38:555–565, 1999

Bower DJ, Chalasani P, Avmons JC: Withdrawal-induced neuroleptic malignant syndrome (letter). Am J Psychiatry 151:451–452, 1994

Bowers MB, Mazure CM, Nelson JC, et al: Lithium in combination with perphenazine: effect on plasma monoamine metabolites. Biol Psychiatry 32:1102–1107, 1992

Branchey M, Charles J, Simpson G: Extrapyramidal side effects in lithium maintenance therapy. Am J Psychiatry 133:444–445, 1976

Brannan SK, Talley BJ, Bowden CL: Sertraline and isocarboxazid cause a serotonin syndrome (letter). J Clin Psychopharmacol 14:144–145, 1994

Brennan D, MacManus M, Howe J, et al: Neuroleptic malignant syndrome without neuroleptics (letter). Br J Psychiatry 152:578–579, 1988

Brodribb TR, Downey M, Gilbar PJ: Efficacy and adverse effects of moclobemide (letter). Lancet 343:475, 1994

Brooks SA: The serotonin syndrome as a learning opportunity (letter). Can J Psychiatry 43:646, 1998

Brown C, Osterloh J: Multiple severe complications from recreational ingestion of MDMA ('Ecstasy') (letter). JAMA 258:780–781, 1987

Brown SJ, Gisolfi CV, Mora F: Temperature regulation and dopaminergic systems in the brain: does the substantia nigra play a role? Brain Res 234:275–286, 1982

Brown TM, Skop BP: Nitroglycerin in the treatment of the serotonin syndrome (letter). Ann Pharmacother 30:191–192, 1996

Brubacher JR, Hoffman RS, Lurin MJ: Serotonin syndrome from venlafaxine-tranylcypromine interaction. Vet Hum Toxicol 38:358–361, 1996

Bruck K: Thermal balance and the regulation of body temperature, in Human Physiology. Edited by Schmidt RF, Thews G. Berlin, Springer-Verlag, 1989, pp 624–644

Brust JC, Hammer JS, Challenor Y, et al: Acute generalized polyneuropathy accompanying lithium poisoning. Ann Neurol 6:360–362, 1979

Bubser M, Schmidt WJ: Injection of apomorphine into the medial prefrontal cortex of the rat increases haloperidol-induced catalepsy. Biol Psychiatry 36:64–67, 1994

Buffat JJ, Rouvier PH, Vasseur C, et al: Fallait-il demembrer le syndrome malin des neuroleptiques? Medecine et Armees 13:767–772, 1985

Bunney WE, Garland-Bunney BL: Mechanism of action of lithium in affective illness: basic and clinical implications, in Psychopharmacology: The Third Generation of Progress. Edited by Meltzer HY, New York, Raven, 1987, pp 553–565

Burch EA, Downs J: Development of neuroleptic malignant syndrome during simultaneous amoxapine treatment and alprazolam discontinuation (letter). J Clin Psychopharmacol 7:55–56, 1987

Burke RE, Fahn S, Mayeux R, et al: Neuroleptic malignant syndrome caused by dopamine-depleting drugs in a patient with Huntington disease. Neurology 31:1022–1026, 1981

Burns RS, Chiueh CC, Markey SP, et al: A primate model of parkinsonism: selective destruction of dopaminergic neurons in the pars compacta of the substantia nigra by N-methyl-4-phenyl-1,2,3,6-tetrahydropyridine. Proc Natl Acad Sci U S A 80:4546–4550, 1983

Burns RS, LeWitt PA, Ebert MH, et al: The clinical syndrome of striatal dopamine deficiency. N Engl J Med 312:1418–1421, 1985

Butzkueven H: A case of serotonin syndrome induced by moclobemide during extreme heat wave (letter). Aust N Z J Med 27:603–604, 1997

Callaway CW, Clark RF: Hyperthermia in psychostimulant overdose. Ann Emerg Med 4:68–76, 1994

Calmeil LF: Dictionnaire de Medecine ou Repertoire General des Sciences. Medicales sous le Rapport Theorique et Practique, 2nd Edition. Paris, Bechet, 1832

Calore EE, Cavaliere MJ, Perez NM, et al: Hyperthermic reaction to haloperidol with rigidity associated with central core disease. Acta Neurologica 16:157–161, 1994

Campkin NT, Davies UM: Another death from Ecstasy (letter). J R Soc Med 85:61, 1992

Cano-Munoz JL, Montejo-Iglesias ML, Yanez-Saez RM, et al: Possible serotonin syndrome following the combined administration of clomipramine and alprazolam (letter). J Clin Psychiatry 56:122, 1995

Cao L, Katz RH: Acute hypernatremia and neuroleptic malignant syndrome in Parkinson disease. Am J Med Sci 318:67–68, 1999

Caroff SN: The neuroleptic malignant syndrome. J Clin Psychiatry 41:79–83, 1980

Caroff SN, Mann SC: Neuroleptic malignant syndrome. Psychopharmacol Bull 24:25–29, 1988

Caroff SN, Mann SC: Neuroleptic malignant syndrome. Med Clin North Am 77: 185–202, 1993

Caroff SN, Rosenberg H, Fletcher J, et al: Malignant hyperthermia susceptibility in neuroleptic malignant syndrome. Anesthesiology 67:20–25, 1987

Caroff SN, Mann SC, Lazarus A, et al: Neuroleptic malignant syndrome: diagnostic issues. Psychiatric Annals 21:130–147, 1991

Caroff SN, Mann SC, Campbell EC: Hyperthermia and neuroleptic malignant syndrome. Anesthesiology Clinics of North America 12:491–512, 1994a

Caroff SN, Mann SC, Sullivan K, et al: Drug-induced hypermetabolic syndromes, in Malignant Hyperthermia: A Genetic Membrane Disease. Edited by Ohnishi ST, Ohnishi T. Boca Raton, FL, CRC Press, 1994b, pp 118–129

Caroff SN, Mann SC, Keck PE Jr: Specific treatment of the neuroleptic malignant syndrome. Biol Psychiatry 44:378–381, 1998a

Caroff SN, Mann SC, McCarthy M, et al: Acute infectious encephalitis complicated by neuroleptic malignant syndrome. J Clin Psychopharmacol 18:349–351, 1998b

Caroff SN, Mann SC, Campbell EC: Atypical antipsychotics and neuroleptic malignant syndrome. Psychiatric Annals 30:314–321, 2000a

Caroff SN, Mann SC, Campbell EC: Risk of fatal heatstroke after hospitalization (letter). Psychiatr Serv 51:938, 2000b

Caroff SN, Mann SC, Keck PE, et al: Residual catatonic state following neuroleptic malignant syndrome. J Clin Psychopharmacol 20:257–259, 2000c

Caroff SN, Mann SC, Campbell EC: Neuroleptic malignant syndrome. Adverse Drug Reaction Bulletin 209:799–802, 2001a

Caroff SN, Mann SC, Gliatto MF, et al: Psychiatric manifestations of acute viral encephalitis. Psychiatric Annals 31:193–204, 2001b

Caroff SN, Rosenberg H, Mann SC, et al: Neuroleptic malignant syndrome in the perioperative setting. American Journal of Anesthesiology 28:387–393, 2001c

Caroff SN, Mann SC, Campbell EC, et al: Movement disorders associated with atypical antipsychotic drugs. J Clin Psychiatry 63 (suppl 4):12–19, 2002

Carroll BT: The universal field hypothesis of catatonia and neuroleptic malignant syndrome. CNS Spectrums 5:26–33, 2000

Carroll BT, Goforth HW: Serum iron and neuroleptic malignant syndrome (letter). Biol Psychiatry 38:776–777, 1995

Carroll BT, Taylor RE: The nondichotomy between lethal catatonia and neuroleptic malignant syndrome (letter). J Clin Psychopharmacol 17:235–238, 1997

Cassidy EM, O'Keane V: Neuroleptic malignant syndrome after venlafaxine. Lancet 355:2164–2165, 2000

Cassidy EM, O'Brien M, Osman MF, et al: Lethal catatonia responding to high-dose olanzapine therapy. J Psychopharmacol 15:302–304, 2001

Casteels-Van Daele M, Van Geet C, Wouters C, et al: Reye syndrome revisited: a descriptive term covering a group of heterogeneous disorders. Eur J Pediatr 159:641–648, 2000

Castillo E, Rubin RT, Holsboer-Trachsler E: Clinical differentiation between lethal catatonia and neuroleptic malignant syndrome. Am J Psychiatry 146:324–328, 1989

Catravas JD, Waters IW: Acute cocaine intoxication in the conscious dog: studies on the mechanism of lethality. J Pharmacol Exp Ther 217:350–356, 1981

Cavanaugh JJ, Finlayson RE: Rhabdomyolysis due to acute dystonic reaction to antipsychotic drugs. J Clin Psychiatry 45:356–357, 1984

Chadwick IS, Curry PD, Linsley A, et al: Ecstasy, 3,4-methylenedioxymethamphetamine, a fatality associated with coagulopathy and hyperthermia (letter). J R Soc Med 84:371, 1991

Chan BS, Graudins A, Whyte IM, et al: Serotonin syndrome resulting from drug interactions. Med J Aust 169:523–525, 1998

Chopra M, Prakash SS, Raguram R: The neuroleptic malignant syndrome: an Indian experience. Compr Psychiatry 40:19–23, 1999

Chrisstoffels J, Thiel JH: Delirium acutum, a potentially fatal condition in the psychiatric hospital. Psychiatria Neurologia Neurochirurgia 73:177–187, 1970

Clark WG, Lipton JM: Drug-related heatstroke. Pharmacol Ther 26:345–388, 1984

Coccaro EF, Siever LJ: Second generation antidepressants: a comparative review. J Clin Pharmacol 25:241–260, 1985

Coffey CE, Ross DR, Ferren EL, et al: Treatment of the "on-off" phenomenon in parkinsonism with lithium carbonate. Ann Neurol 12:375–379, 1982

Cogen FC, Rigg G, Simmons JL, et al: Phencyclidine-associated acute rhabdomyolysis. Ann Intern Med 88:210–212, 1978

Cohen S, Fligner CL, Raisys VA, et al: A case of non-neuroleptic malignant syndrome. J Clin Psychiatry 48:287–288, 1987

Cohen WJ, Cohen NH: Lithium carbonate, haloperidol, and irreversible brain damage. JAMA 230:1283–1287, 1974

Coorey AN, Wenck DJ: Venlafaxine overdose (letter). Med J Aust 163:523, 1998

Coplan JD, Gorman JM: Detectable levels of fluoxetine metabolites after discontinuation: an unexpected serotonin syndrome (letter). Am J Psychiatry 150:837, 1993

Corkeron MA: Serotonin syndrome—a potentially fatal complication of antidepressant therapy. Med J Aust 163:481–482, 1995

Cox B, Lee TF: Location of receptors mediating hypothermia after injection of dopamine agonists in rats. Br J Pharmacol 59:467–468, 1977

Cox B, Lee TF: Further evidence for a physiological role for hypothalamic dopamine in thermoregulation in the rat. J Physiol (Lond) 300:7–17, 1980

Cox B, Tha SJ: The role of dopamine and noradrenaline in temperature control of normal and reserpine-pretreated mice. J Pharm Pharmacol 27:242–247, 1975

Cox B, Kerwin R, Lee TF: Dopamine receptors in the central thermoregulatory pathways of the rat. J Physiol (Lond) 282:471–483, 1978

Cox B, Kerwin RW, Lee TF, et al: A dopamine-5-hydroxytryptamine link in the hypothalamic pathways, which mediate heat loss in the rat. J Physiol (Lond) 303: 9–21, 1980

Crandall CG, Vongputanasin W, Victor RG: Mechanism of cocaine-induced hyperthermia in humans. Ann Intern Med 136:785–791, 2002

Crews EL, Carpenter AE: Lithium-induced aggravation of tardive dyskinesia. Am J Psychiatry 134:933, 1977

Cryan JF, Harkin A, Naughton M, et al: Characterization of D-fenfluramine-induced hypothermia: evidence for multiple sites of action. Eur J Pharmacol 390:275–285, 2000

Cullumbine H, Miles S: The effect of atropine sulphate on men exposed to warm environments. Quarterly Journal of Experimental Physiology 41:162–179, 1956

Cummings JL: Frontal-subcortical circuits and human behavior. Arch Neurol 50:873–880, 1993

Cunningham MA, Darby DG, Donnan GA: Controlled-release delivery of L-DOPA associated with nonfatal hyperthermia, rigidity and autonomic dysfunction. Neurology 41:942–943, 1991

Curzon G, Ettlinger G, Cole M, et al: The biochemical, behavioral and neurological effects of high L-tryptophan intake in the rhesus monkey. Neurology 12:431–438, 1963

Daniels RJ: Serotonin syndrome due to venlafaxine overdose. J Accid Emerg Med 15:333–334, 1998

Daras M, Kakkouras L, Tuchman AJ, et al: Rhabdomyolysis and hyperthermia after cocaine abuse: a variant of the neuroleptic malignant syndrome? Acta Neurol Scand 92:161–165, 1995

Dardennes RM, Even C, Ballon N, et al: Serotonin syndrome caused by a clomipramine-moclobemide interaction (letter). J Clin Psychiatry 59:382–383, 1998

Davis JM, Janicak PG, Sakkas P, et al: Electroconvulsive therapy in the treatment of the neuroleptic malignant syndrome. Convulsive Therapy 7:111–120, 1991

Davis JM, Caroff SN, Mann SC: Treatment of neuroleptic malignant syndrome. Psychiatric Annals 30:325–331, 2000

Davis WM, Logston DH, Hickenbottom JP: Antagonism of acute amphetamine intoxication by haloperidol and propranolol. Toxicol Appl Pharmacol 29:397–403, 1974

Dekleva KB, Husain MM: Sporadic encephalitis lethargica: a case treated successfully with ECT. J Neuropsychiatry Clin Neurosci 7:237–239, 1995

Delay J, Deniker P: Drug-induced extrapyramidal syndromes, in Handbook of Clinical Neurology, Vol 6: Diseases of the Basal Ganglia. Edited by Vinken PJ, Bruyn GW. Amsterdam, North-Holland, 1968, pp 248–266

Delay J, Pichot P, Lemperiere T, et al: Un neuroleptique majeur non phenothiazine et non reserpinique, l'haloperidol, dans le traitement des psychoses. Annales Médico-Psychologiques (Paris) 118:145–152, 1960

Demetriou S, Fucek FR, Domino EF: Lack of effect of acute and chronic lithium on chlorpromazine plasma and brain levels in the rat. Common Psychopharmacology 3:17–24, 1979

Demirkiran M, Jankovic J, Dean JM: Ecstasy intoxication: an overlap between serotonin syndrome and neuroleptic malignant syndrome. Clin Neuropharmacol 19:157–164, 1996

Denborough MA, Hopkinson KC: Dantrolene and "ecstasy." Med J Aust 166:165–166, 1997

Deng MZ, Chen GQ, Phillips MR: Neuroleptic malignant syndrome in 12 of 9,792 Chinese inpatients exposed to neuroleptics: a prospective study. Am J Psychiatry 147:1149–1155, 1990

Denton PH, Borrelli VM, Edwards NV: Dangers of monoamine oxidase inhibitors. BMJ 2:1752–1753, 1962

Derby IM: Manic-depressive "exhaustive" deaths. Psychiatr Q 7:436–449, 1933

DeReuck J, Van Aken J, Van Landegem W, et al: Positron emission tomographic studies of changes in cerebral blood flow and oxygen metabolism in neuroleptic malignant syndrome. Eur Neurol 31:1–6, 1991

De Roij TAJM, Frens J, Barker J, et al: Thermoregulatory effects of intraventricularly injected dopamine in the goat. Eur J Pharmacol 43:1–7, 1977

De Roij TAJM, Bligh J, Smith CA, et al: Comparison of the thermoregulatory responses to intracerebroventricularly injected dopamine and noradrenaline in the sheep. Naunyn Schmiedebergs Arch Pharmacol 303:263–269, 1978a

De Roij TAJM, Frens J, Woutersen-Van Nijanten F, et al: Comparison of the thermoregulatory responses to intracerebroventricularly injected dopamine, noradrenaline and 5-hydroxytryptamine in the goat. Eur J Pharmacol 49:395–405, 1978b

Destee A, Montagne B, Rousseaux M, et al: Incidents et accidents des neuroleptiques (110 hospitalisations en neurologie). Lille Medical 25:291–295, 1980

Deuschl G, Oepen G, Hermle L, et al: Neuroleptic malignant syndrome: observations on altered consciousness. Pharmacopsychiatry 20:168–170, 1987

Deutch AY, Bourdelais AJ, Zahm DS: The nucleus accumbens core and shell: accumbal compartments and their functional attributes, in Limbic Motor Circuits and Neuropsychiatry. Edited by Kalivas PW, Barnes CD. Boca Raton, FL, CRC Press, 1993, pp 163–175

Diamond C, Pepper BJ, Diamond ML, et al: Serotonin syndrome induced by transitioning from phenelzine to venlafaxine: four patient reports. Neurology 51:274–276, 1998

Dilsaver SC: Lithium down-regulates nicotinic receptors in skeletal muscle: cause of lithium-associated myasthenic syndrome (letter)? J Clin Psychopharmacol 7:369–370, 1987

Dingemanse J, Wallnofer A, Gieschke R, et al: Pharmacokinetic and pharmacodynamic interactions between fluoxetine and moclobemide in the investigation of development of serotonin syndrome. Clin Pharmacol Ther 63:403–413, 1998

Domino EF: Neurobiology of phencyclidine (Sernyl): a drug with an unusual spectrum of pharmacologic activity. International Journal of Neurobiology 6:303–347, 1964

Donaldson IM, Cunningham J: Persisting neurologic sequelae of lithium carbonate therapy. Arch Neurol 40:747–751, 1983

Downey GP, Rosenberg M, Caroff S, et al: Neuroleptic malignant syndrome. Am J Med 77:338–340, 1984

Downey RJ, Downey JA, Newhouse E, et al: Fatal hyperthermia in a quadriplegic man: possible evidence of peripheral action of haloperidol in neuroleptic malignant syndrome. Chest 101:1728–1730, 1992

Draper DD, Rothschild MF, Beitz DC, et al: Age and genotype dependent differences in catecholamine concentrations in the porcine caudate nucleus. Exp Gerontol 19:377–381, 1984

Dursun SM, Mathew VM, Reveley MA: Toxic serotonin syndrome after fluoxetine plus carbamazepine (letter). Lancet 342:442–443, 1993

Dursun SM, Burke JG, Reveley MA: Toxic serotonin syndrome or extrapyramidal side-effects (letter)? Br J Psychiatry 52:401–402, 1995

Ebert D, Albert R, May A, et al: The serotonin syndrome and psychosis-like side-effects of fluvoxamine clinical use—an estimation of incidence. Eur Neuropsychopharmacol 7:71–74, 1997

Egberts AC, Ter Borgh J, Brodie-Meijer CC: Serotonin syndrome attributed to tramadol addition to paroxetine therapy. Int Clin Psychopharmacol 12:181–182, 1997

Elizur A, Shopsin B, Gershon S, et al: Intra/extracellular lithium ratios and clinical course in affective states. Clin Pharmacol Ther 13:947–952, 1972

Elizur A, Graff E, Steiner M, et al: Intra/extra red cell lithium and electrolyte distributions as correlates of neurotoxic reactions during lithium therapy, in The Impact of Biology on Modern Psychiatry. Edited by Gershon ES, Belmaker RH, Kety SS, et al. New York, Plenum, 1977, pp 55–64

Engel J, Berggren U: Effects of lithium on behavior and central monoamines. Acta Psychiatr Scand 61:133–142, 1980

Eroglu L, Hizal A, Koyuncuogli H: The effect of long-term concurrent administration of chlorpromazine and lithium on the striatal and frontal cortical dopamine metabolism in rats. Psychopharmacology 73:84–86, 1981

Evans DL, Garner BW: Neurotoxicity at therapeutic lithium levels (letter). Am J Psychiatry 136:1481–1482, 1979

Fabre S, Gervais C, Manuel C, et al: [Toxic syndrome induced by neuroleptics: report of 7 cases]. Encephale 3:321–326, 1977

Fadda F, Serra G, Argiolas A, et al: Effect of lithium on 3, 4-dihydroxy-phenylacetic acid (DOPAC) concentrations in different brain areas of rats. Pharmacological Research Communications 12:689–693, 1980

Faunt JE, Crocker AD: The effects of selective dopamine receptor agonists and antagonists on body temperature. Eur J Pharmacol 133:243–247, 1987

Feibel JH, Schiffer RB: Sympathoadrenomedullary hyperactivity in the neuroleptic malignant syndrome: a case report. Am J Psychiatry 138:1115–1116, 1981

Feigenbaum JJ, Yanai J: Implications of dopamine agonist-induced hypothermia following increased density of dopamine receptors in the mouse. Neuropharmacology 24:735–741, 1985

Ferrer-Dufol A, Perez-Arados C, Murillo EC: Fatal serotonin syndrome caused by moclobemide-clomipramine overdose (letter). Clin Toxicol 36:31–32, 1998

Ferro FM, Janiri L, De Bonis C, et al: Clinical outcome and psychoendocrinological findings in a case of lethal catatonia. Biol Psychiatry 30:197–200, 1991

Figa-Talamanca L, Gualandi C, DiMeo L, et al: Hyperthermia after discontinuance of levodopa and bromocriptine therapy: impaired dopamine receptors a possible cause. Neurology 35:258–261, 1985

Fink M: Neuroleptic malignant syndrome and catatonia: one entity or two? Biol Psychiatry 39:1–4, 1996

Fink M: Catatonia: syndrome or schizophrenia subtype? Recognition and treatment. J Neural Transm 108:637–644, 2001

Finkelman I, Stephens WM: Heat regulation in dementia praecox. Am J Psychiatry 92:1185–1189, 1936

Fischer P: Serotonin syndrome in the elderly after antidepressive monotherapy. J Clin Psychopharmacol 15:440–442, 1995

Fischman MW: Cocaine and the amphetamines, in Psychopharmacology: The Third Generation of Progress. Edited by Meltzer HY. New York, Raven, 1987, pp 1543–1553

Fisher KJ, Greiner A: "Acute lethal catatonia" treated by hypothermia. Canadian Medical Association Journal 82:630–634, 1960

FitzSimmons CR, Metha S: Serotonin syndrome caused by overdose with paroxetine and moclobemide. J Accid Emerg Med 16:293–295, 1999

Fjalland B: Antagonism of apomorphine-induced hyperthermia in MAOI-pretreated rabbits as a sensitive model of neuroleptic activity. Psychopharmacology 63:119–123, 1979

Fleischhacker WW, Unterweger B, Kane JM, et al: The neuroleptic malignant syndrome and its differentiation from lethal catatonia. Acta Psychiatr Scand 81:3–5, 1990

Flemenbaum A: Lithium inhibition of norepinephrine and dopamine receptors. Biol Psychiatry 12:536–572, 1977

Flyckt L, Borg J, Borg K, et al: Muscle biopsy, macro EMG, and clinical characteristics in patients with schizophrenia. Biol Psychiatry 47:991–999, 2000

Forsman A, Ohman R: Studies on serum protein binding of haloperidol. Curr Ther Res Clin Exp 21:245–255, 1977

Foti ME, Pies RW: Lithium carbonate and tardive dyskinesia (letter). J Clin Psychopharmacol 6:325–326, 1986

Francis A, Petrides G: Similarity of catatonia and NMS. Paper presented at the 151st annual meeting of the American Psychiatric Association, Toronto, Ontario, Canada, May 30–June 4, 1998

Francis A, Chondragivi S, Rizvi S, et al: Is lorazepam a treatment for neuroleptic malignant syndrome? CNS Spectrums 5:54–57, 2000

Francois B, Marquet P, Desachy A, et al: Serotonin syndrome due to an overdose of moclobemide and clomipramine: a potentially life-threatening association. Intensive Care Med 23:122–124, 1997

Freeman W, Dumoff E: Cerebellar syndrome following heatstroke. Arch Neurol Psychiatry 51:67–72, 1944

Frey HH: Hyperthermia induced by amphetamine, p-chloroamphetamine and fenfluramine in the rat. Pharmacology 13:163–176, 1975

Fricchione GL: Neuroleptic catatonia and its relationship to psychogenic catatonia. Biol Psychiatry 20:304–313, 1985

Fricchione G, Kaufman LD, Fink M: Electroconvulsive therapy and cyclophosphamide in combination for severe neuropsychiatric lupus with catatonia. Am J Med 88:442–443, 1990

Fricchione G, Bush G, Fozdar M, et al: Recognition and treatment of the catatonic syndrome. Journal of Intensive Care Medicine 12:135–147, 1997

Fricchione G, Mann SC, Caroff SN: Catatonia, lethal catatonia, and neuroleptic malignant syndrome. Psychiatric Annals 31:347–355, 2000

Friedman E, Gershon S: Effect of lithium on brain dopamine. Nature 243:520–521, 1973

Friedman JH, Feinberg SS, Feldman RG: A neuroleptic malignant-like syndrome due to levodopa therapy withdrawal. JAMA 254:2792–2794, 1985

Friedman SA, Hirsch SE: Extreme hyperthermia after LSD ingestion. JAMA 217: 1549–1550, 1971

Fuchs F: Thermal inactivation of the calcium regulatory mechanism of human skeletal muscle actomyosin: a possible contributing factor in the rigidity of malignant hyperthermia. Anesthesiology 42:584–589, 1975

Gabuzda DH, Frankenburg FR: Fever caused by lithium in a patient with neuroleptic malignant syndrome (letter). J Clin Psychopharmacol 7:283–284, 1987

Gardner DM, Lynd LD: Sumatriptan contraindications and the serotonin syndrome. Ann Pharmacother 32:33–38, 1998

Gary NE, Saidi P: Methamphetamine intoxication: a speedy new treatment. Am J Med 64:537–540, 1978

Geiduschek J, Cohen SA, Khan A, et al: Repeated anesthesia for a patient with neuroleptic malignant syndrome. Anesthesiology 68:134–137, 1988

Geisler A, Klysner R: Combined effect of lithium and flupenthixol on striatal adenylate cyclase (letter). Lancet 1:430–431, 1977

Gelenberg AJ: The catatonic syndrome. Lancet 1:1339–1341, 1976

Gelenberg AJ, Bellinghausen B, Wojcik JD, et al: A prospective survey of neuroleptic malignant syndrome in a short-term psychiatric hospital. Am J Psychiatry 145:517–518, 1988

Gelenberg AJ, Bellinghausen B, Wojik JD, et al: Patients with neuroleptic malignant syndrome histories: what happens when they are rehospitalized? J Clin Psychiatry 50:178–180, 1989

Geller B, Greydanus DE: Haloperidol-induced comatose state with hyperthermia and rigidity in adolescence: two case reports with a literature review. J Clin Psychiatry 40:102–103, 1979

George TP, Godleski LS: Possible serotonin syndrome with trazodone addition to fluoxetine (letter). Biol Psychiatry 39:384–385, 1996

Gerlach J, Thorsen K, Munkuud I: Effect of lithium in neuroleptic-induced tardive dyskinesia compared with placebo in a double-blind cross-over trial. Pharmakopsychiatrie Neuropsychopharmakologie 8:51–56, 1975

Gerra G, Zaimovic A, Ferri M, et al: Long-lasting effects of 3,4-methylenedioxymethamphetamine (Ecstasy) on serotonin system function in humans. Biol Psychiatry 47:127–136, 2000

Gerson S, Baldessarini RJ: Motor effects of serotonin in the central nervous system. Life Sci 27:1435–1451, 1980

Gertz HJ, Schmidt LG: Low melanin content of substantia nigra in a case of neuroleptic malignant syndrome. Pharmacopsychiatry 24:93–95, 1991

Ghadirian AM, Nair NPV, Schwartz G: Effect of lithium and neuroleptic combination on lithium transport, blood pressure, and weight in bipolar patients. Biol Psychiatry 26:139–144, 1989

Gibb WRG: Neuroleptic malignant syndrome in striatonigral degeneration. Br J Psychiatry 153:254–255, 1988

Gill JR, Hayes JA, deSonza IS, et al: Ecstasy (MDMA) deaths in New York City: a case series and review of the literature. J Forensic Sci 47:121–126, 2002

Gillman PK: Possible serotonin syndrome with moclobemide and pethidine (letter). Med J Aust 162:554, 1995

Gillman PK: Successful treatment of serotonin syndrome with chlorpromazine (letter). Med J Aust 165:345–346, 1996

Gillman PK: Ecstasy, serotonin syndrome and the treatment of hyperpyrexia (letter). Med J Aust 167:109, 1997a

Gillman PK: Serotonin syndrome—clomipramine too soon after moclobemide? Int Clin Psychopharmacol 12:339–342, 1997b

Gingrich JA, Rudnick-Levin F, Almeida C, et al: Cocaine and catatonia (letter). Am J Psychiatry 155:1629, 1998

Ginsberg MD, Hertzman M, Schmidt-Nawara WW: Amphetamine intoxication with coagulopathy, hyperthermia, and reversible renal failure. Ann Intern Med 73:81–85, 1970

Girke W, Krebs FA, Muller-Oerlinghausen B: Effects of lithium on electromyographic recordings in man. International Pharmacopsychiatry 10:24–36, 1975

Giroud M, Buffat JJ, Le Bris H, et al: Unsuffisance respiratoire aigue et traitement psychiatrique au long cours (a propos de onze observations). Lyon Medicine 239:251–255, 1978

Gitlin MJ: Venlafaxine, monoamine oxidase inhibitors, and the serotonin syndrome (letter). J Clin Psychopharmacol 17:66–67, 1997

Glennon RA: Do classical hallucinations act as $5\text{-}HT_2$ agonists or antagonists? Neuropsychopharmacology 3:509–517, 1990

Goeke JE, Hagan DS, Goelzer SL, et al: Lethal catatonia complicated by the development of neuroleptic malignant syndrome in a middle-aged female. Crit Care Med 19:1445–1448, 1991

Goforth HW, Carroll BT: The overlap of neuroleptic malignant syndrome (NMS) and catatonic diagnoses (abstract). J Neuropsychiatry Clin Neurosci 7:402, 1995

Gold MS, Tabrah H, Frost-Pineda K: Psychopharmacology of MDMA (Ecstasy). Psychiatric Annals 31:675–681, 2001

Goldberg RJ, Huk M: Serotonin syndrome from trazodone and buspirone (letter). Psychosomatics 33:235–236, 1992

Goldman SA: FDA Medwatch report: lithium and neuroleptics in combination: the spectrum of neurotoxicity. Psychopharmacol Bull 32:299–309, 1996a

Goldman SA: Lithium and neuroleptics in combination: is there enhancement of neurotoxicity leading to permanent sequellae? J Clin Pharmacol 36:951–962, 1996b

Goldney RD, Spence ND: Safety of the combination of lithium and neuroleptic drugs. Am J Psychiatry 143:882–884, 1986

Gordon PH, Frucht SJ: Neuroleptic malignant syndrome in advanced Parkinson's disease. Mov Disord 16:960–974, 2001

Gorodetzky CW, Isbell H: A comparison of 2,3-dihydrolysergic acid diethylamide with LSD-25. Psychopharmacologia 6:229–233, 1964

Gottlieb JS, Linder S: Body temperature of persons with schizophrenia and of normal subjects. Archives of Neurology and Psychiatry 33:775–785, 1935

Gowing LR, Henry-Edwards SM, Irvine RT, et al: The health effects of ecstasy: a literature review. Drug and Alcohol Review 21:53–63, 2002

Graber MA, Hoehns TB, Perry PJ: Sertraline-phenelzine drug interaction: a serotonin syndrome reaction. Ann Pharmacother 28:732–735, 1994

Grahame-Smith DG: Inhibitory effect of chlorpromazine on the syndrome of hyperactivity produced by L-tryptophan or 5-methoxy-N, N-dimethyltryptamine in rats treated with a monoamine oxidase inhibitor. Br J Pharmacol 43:856–864, 1971

Grant R: Neuroleptic malignant syndrome (letter). BMJ 288:1690, 1984

Grantham J, Neel W, Brown RW: Reversal of imipramine-monoamine oxidase inhibitor induced toxicity with chlorpromazine. Journal of the Kansas Medical Society 65:279–280, 1964

Graudins A, Stearman A, Chan B: Treatment of serotonin syndrome with cyproheptadine. J Emerg Med 16:615–619, 1998

Green AR, Cross AJ, Goodwin GM: Review of the pharmacology and clinical pharmacology of 3,4-methylene dioxymethamphetamine (MDMA or "ecstasy"). Psychopharmacology 119:247–260, 1995

Greenberg LB, Gujavarty K: The neuroleptic malignant syndrome: review and report of three cases. Compr Psychiatry 26:63–70, 1985

Grigg JR: Neuroleptic malignant syndrome and malignant hyperthermia (letter). Am J Psychiatry 145:1175, 1988

Growe GA, Crayton JW, Klass DB, et al: Lithium in chronic schizophrenia. Am J Psychiatry 136:454–455, 1979

Grunhaus L, Sancovici S, Rimon R: Neuroleptic malignant syndrome due to depot fluphenazine. J Clin Psychiatry 40:99–100, 1979

Gudelsky GA, Koenig JI, Meltzer HY: Thermoregulatory responses to serotonin (5-HT) receptor stimulation in the rat. Neuropharmacology 25:1307–1313, 1986

Gurrera RJ: Sympathoadrenal hyperactivity and the etiology of neuroleptic malignant syndrome. Am J Psychiatry 156:169–180, 1999

Gurrera RJ, Chang SS: Thermoregulatory dysfunction in neuroleptic malignant syndrome. Biol Psychiatry 39:207–212, 1996

Gurrera RJ, Romero JA: Enzyme elevations in the neuroleptic malignant syndrome. Biol Psychiatry 34:634–640, 1993

Gurrera RJ, Chang SS, Romero JA: A comparison of diagnostic criteria for neuroleptic malignant syndrome. J Clin Psychiatry 53:56–62, 1992

Guyton AC, Hall JE: Textbook of Medical Physiology. Philadelphia, PA, WB Saunders, 2000

Guze BH, Baxter LR Jr: The serotonin syndrome: case responsive to propranolol (letter). J Clin Psychopharmacol 6:119–120, 1986

Hafner H, Kasper S: Akute lebensbedrohliche Katatonie: Epidemiologische und Klinische Befunde. Nervenzart 53:385–394, 1982

Haggerty JJ Jr, Bentsen BS, Gillette GM: Neuroleptic malignant syndrome superimposed on tardive dyskinesia. Br J Psychiatry 150:104–105, 1987

Hamilton S, Malone K: Serotonin syndrome during treatment with paroxetine and risperidone (letter). J Clin Psychopharmacol 20:103–104, 2000

Hansen HE, Amdisen A: Lithium intoxication: report of 23 cases and review of 100 cases from the literature. Q J Med 47:123–144, 1978

Harris M, Nora L, Tanner OM: Neuroleptic malignant syndrome responsive to carbidopa/levodopa: support for a dopaminergic hypothesis. Clin Neuropharmacol 10:186–189, 1987

Harsch HH: Neuroleptic malignant syndrome: physiological and laboratory findings in a series of nine cases. J Clin Psychiatry 48:328–333, 1987

Hasan S, Buckley P: Novel antipsychotics and the neuroleptic malignant syndrome: a review and critique. Am J Psychiatry 155:1113–1116, 1998

Hayashi K, Chihara E, Scana T, et al: Clinical features of neuroleptic malignant syndrome in basal ganglia disease. Anaesthesia 48:499–502, 1993

Hegadoren KM, Baker GB, Bourin M: 3,4-Methylenedioxy analogues of amphetamine: defining the risks to humans. Neurosci Biobehav Rev 23:539–553, 1999

Hegerl U, Bottlender R, Gallinant J, et al: The Serotonin Syndrome Scale: first results on validity. Eur Arch Psychiatry Clin Neurosci 248:96–103, 1998

Heh CW, Herrera J, DeMet E, et al: Neuroleptic-induced hypothermia associated with amelioration of psychosis in schizophrenia. Neuropharmacology 1:149–156, 1988

Heikkila RE, Sonsalla PK, Kindt MV, et al: MPTP and animal models of parkinsonism, in Handbook of Parkinson's Disease. Edited by Koller WC. New York, Marcel Dekker, 1987, pp 267–279

Heisler MA, Guidry JR, Arnecke B: Serotonin syndrome induced by administration of venlafaxine and phenelzine (letter). Ann Pharmacother 30:84, 1996

Henderson A, Longdon P: Fulminant metoclopramide induced neuroleptic malignant syndrome rapidly responsive to dantrolene. Aust N Z J Med 21:742–743, 1991

Henderson VW, Wooten GF: Neuroleptic malignant syndrome: a pathogenetic role for dopamine receptor blockade? Neurology 31:132–137, 1981

Henry JA: Metabolic consequences of drug misuse. Br J Anaesth 85:136–142, 2000

Henry JA, Jeffreys KJ, Dawling S: Toxicity and deaths from 3,4-methylenedioxymethamphetamine ('ecstasy'). Lancet 340:384–387, 1992

Henry P, Barat M, Bourgeois M: Syndrome malin mortel succedent a une injection d'emblee d'oenanthate de fluphenazine. Presse Med 79:1350, 1971

Hermesh H, Aizenberg D, Lapidot M: Risk of malignant hyperthermia among patients with neuroleptic malignant syndrome and their families. Am J Psychiatry 145:1431–1434, 1988

Hermesh H, Aizenberg D, Weizman A, et al: Risk for definite neuroleptic malignant syndrome: a prospective study in 223 consecutive inpatients. Br J Psychiatry 161:254–257, 1992

Hermesh H, Manor I, Aizenberg D, et al: Serum muscle enzyme levels and WBC count: risk factors for neuroleptic malignant syndrome? Eur Neuropsychopharmacol 6 (suppl 4):114–119, 1996

Hermesh H, Shiloh R, Epistein Y, et al: Heat intolerance in patients with chronic schizophrenia maintained with antipsychotic drugs. Am J Psychiatry 157:1327–1329, 2000

Hernandez AF, Montero MN, Pla A, et al: Fatal moclobemide overdose or death caused by serotonin syndrome? J Forensic Sci 40:128–130, 1995

Herzlich BC, Arsura EL, Pagala M, et al: Rhabdomyolysis related to cocaine abuse. Ann Intern Med 109:335–336, 1988

Hesketh JE, Nicolaou NM, Arbuthnott GW, et al: The effect of chronic lithium administration on dopamine metabolism in rat striatum. Psychopharmacology 56:163–166, 1978

Hewick DS, Murray N: Red blood cell levels and lithium toxicity (letter). Lancet 2:473, 1976

Hilton SE, Maradit H, Moller HJ: Serotonin syndrome and drug combinations: focus on MAOI and RIMA. Eur Arch Psychiatry Clin Neurosci 247:113–119, 1997

Himmelhoch JM, Neil JF, May SJ, et al: Age, dementia, dyskinesias and lithium response. Am J Psychiatry 137:941–945, 1980

Hjorth S, Carlsson A: In vivo binding, neurochemical and functional studies with the dopamine D-1 receptor antagonist SCH 23390. J Neural Transm 72:83–97, 1988

Hodgman MJ, Martin TG, Krenzelok EP: Serotonin syndrome due to venlafaxine and maintenance tranylcypromine therapy. Hum Exp Toxicol 16:14–17, 1997

Hoes MJ, Zeijpveld JH: Mirtazapine as treatment for serotonin syndrome (letter). Pharmacopsychiatry 29:81, 1996

Hon CA, Landers DF, Platts AA: Effects of neuroleptic agents on rat skeletal muscle contracture in-vitro. Anesth Analg 72:194–202, 1991

Horn E, Lach B, Lapierre Y, et al: Hypothalamic pathology in the neuroleptic malignant syndrome. Am J Psychiatry 145:617–620, 1988

Horowitz BZ, Mullins ME: Cyproheptadine for serotonin syndrome in an accidental pediatric sertraline ingestion. Pediatr Emerg Care 15:325–327, 1999

Huber G: Zur nosologischen Differenzierung lebensbedrohlicher katatoner Psychosen. Schweizer Archiv fur Neurologie und Neurochir Psychiatrie 74:216–244, 1954

Huckle P, Kellam A, Williams P, et al: Do cases of neuroleptic malignant syndrome cluster? Irish Journal of Psychological Medicine 10:28–29, 1993

Insel TR, Roy BF, Cohen RM, et al: Possible development of the serotonin syndrome in man. Am J Psychol 139:954–955, 1982

Ito T, Shibata K, Watanabe A, et al: Neuroleptic malignant syndrome following withdrawal of amantadine in a patient with influenza A encephalopathy (letter). Eur J Pediatr 160:401, 2001

Itoh H, Ohtsuka N, Ogita K, et al: Malignant neuroleptic syndrome: its present status in Japan and clinical problems. Folia Psychiatrica et Neurologica Japonica 31:559–576, 1977

Itoh M, Nakano E, Ieshima A, et al: Neuroleptic malignant syndrome in striatonigral degeneration. Pediatr Neurol 13:255–256, 1995

Ivanusa A, Hecimovic H, Demarin V: Serotonin syndrome. Neuropsychiatry Neuropsychol Behav Neurol 10:209–212, 1997

Iwahashi K: CYP2D6 genotype and possible susceptibility to the neuroleptic malignant syndrome. Biol Psychiatry 36:780–782, 1994

Iwahashi K, Yoshihara E, Nakamura K, et al: CYP2D6 HhaI genotype and the neuroleptic malignant syndrome. Neuropsychobiology 39:33–37, 1999

Iwasaki Y, Kinoshita M, Ikeda K, et al: Iron, Parkinson's disease, and neuroleptic malignant syndrome (letter). Neurology 42:1845, 1992

Iwuagwu CU, Bonomo RA: Neuroleptic malignant-like syndrome in an elderly patient caused by abrupt withdrawal of tolcapone, a catechol-O-methyl transferase inhibitor (letter). Am J Med 108:517–518, 2000

Izzo KL, Brody R: Rehabilitation in lithium toxicity: case report. Arch Phys Med Rehabil 66:779–782, 1985

Jackson DM, Wikstrom H, Liao Y: Is clozapine an (partial) agonist at both D-1 and D-2 receptors (letter)? Psychopharmacology 138:213–214, 1998

Jacobs BL: An animal behavioral model for studying central serotonergic synapses. Life Sci 19:777–785, 1976

Jacobs BL, Klemfuss H: Brain stem and spinal cord mediation of a serotonergic behavioral syndrome. Brain Res 100:450–457, 1975

Jahn D, Greving H: Untersuchung uber die korperlichen Storungen bei katatonen Stuporen und der todlichen Katatonie. Archiv fur Psychiatrie und Nervenkrankheiten 105:105–120, 1936

Jahr JS, Pisto JD, Gitlin MC, et al: The serotonin syndrome in a patient receiving sertraline after an ankle block. Anesth Analg 79:189–191, 1994

Janati A, Webb T: Successful treatment of neuroleptic malignant syndrome with bromocriptine. South Med J 79:1567–1571, 1986

Jauss M, Krack P, Franz M, et al: Imaging of dopamine receptors with ^{123}I-Iodo-benzamide single-photon emission-computed tomography in neuroleptic malignant syndrome. Mov Disord 11:726–728, 1996

Jefferson JW, Greist JH: Haloperidol and lithium: their combined use and the issue of their compatibility, in Haloperidol Update: 1958–1980. Edited by Ayd FJ Jr. Baltimore, MD, Ayd Medical Communications, 1980, pp 73–82

Jefferson JW, Greist JH, Ackerman DL, et al: Lithium Encyclopedia for Clinical Practice, 2nd Edition. Washington, DC, American Psychiatric Press, 1987

Jenner P, Marsden CD: Dopamine neurone destruction in human and animal parkinsonism, in Dopaminergic Systems and Their Regulation. Edited by Woodruff GH, Poat JA, Roberts PJ. Deerfield Beach, FL, VCH Publishers, 1986, pp 243–259

Jennings AE, Levey AS, Harrington JT: Amoxapine-associated acute renal failure. Arch Intern Med 143:1525–1527, 1983

Joffe RT, Sokolov ST: Co-administration of fluoxetine and sumatriptan: the Canadian experience. Acta Psychiatr Scand 95:551–552, 1997

John L, Perreault MM, Tao T, et al: Serotonin syndrome associated with nefazodone and paroxetine. Ann Emerg Med 29:287–289, 1997

Johnels B, Wallin L, Walinder J: Extrapyramidal side effects of lithium treatment (letter). BMJ 2:642, 1976

Johnson J, Lucey PA: Encephalitis lethargica: a contemporary cause of catatonic stupor. Br J Psychiatry 151:550–552, 1987

Jones EM, Dawson A: Neuroleptic malignant syndrome: a case report with postmortem brain and muscle pathology. J Neurol Neurosurg Psychiatry 52:1006–1009, 1989

Jones ST, Liang AP, Kilbourne EM, et al: Morbidity and mortality associated with the July 1980 heat wave in St. Louis and Kansas City, Mo. JAMA 247:3327–3331, 1982

Juhl RP, Tsuang MT, Perry PJ: Concomitant administration of haloperidol and lithium carbonate in acute mania. Diseases of the Nervous System 38:675–676, 1977

Julien J, Vallat JM, Laguerry A: Myopathy and cerebellar syndrome during acute poisoning with lithium carbonate (letter). Muscle Nerve 2:240, 1979

Jurkat-Rott K, McCarthy T, Lehmann-Horn F: Genetics and pathogenesis of malignant hyperthermia. Muscle Nerve 23:4–17, 2000

Jus A, Villanueva A, Gautier G, et al: Deanol, lithium, and placebo in the treatment of tardive dyskinesia. Neuropsychobiology 4:140–149, 1978

Kapur S, Remington G: Serotonin-dopamine interaction and its relevance to schizophrenia. Am J Psychiatry 153:466–476, 1996

Kapur S, Seeman P: Does fast dissociation from the dopamine D-2 receptor explain the action of atypical antipsychotics? A new hypothesis. Am J Psychiatry 158:360–369, 2001

Kapur S, Zipursky RB, Remington G: Clinical and theoretical implications of 5-HT 2 and D-2 receptor occupancy of clozapine, risperidone, and olanzapine in schizophrenia. Am J Psychiatry 156:286–293, 1999

Kato T, Yamawaki S: A pharmacological study of veratrine-induced hyperthermia in the rat: a model of neuroleptic malignant syndrome. Hiroshima J Med Sci 38:173–181, 1989

Kaufmann CA, Wyatt RJ: Neuroleptic malignant syndrome, in Psychopharmacology: The Third Generation of Progress. Edited by Meltzer HY. New York, Raven, 1987, pp 1421–1430

Kawanishi C, Hanihara T, Shimoda Y, et al: Lack of association between neuroleptic malignant syndrome and polymorphisms in the 5-HT$_{1A}$ and 5-HT$_{2A}$ receptor genes. Am J Psychiatry 155:1275–1277, 1998a

Kawanishi C, Shimoda Y, Fujimaki J, et al: Mutation involving cytochrome P450 II D6 in two Japanese patients with neuroleptic malignant syndrome. J Neurol Sci 160:102–104, 1998b

Kawanishi C, Furuno T, Onishi H, et al: Lack of association in Japanese patients between neuroleptic malignant syndrome and a debrisoquine 4-hydroxylase genotype with low enzyme activity. Psychiatr Genet 10:145–147, 2000

Keck PE Jr, Arnold LM: Serotonin syndrome. Psychiatric Annals 30:333–343, 2000

Keck PE Jr, Pope HG, McElroy SL: Frequency and presentation of neuroleptic malignant syndrome: a prospective study. Am J Psychiatry 144:1344–1346, 1987

Keck PE Jr, Pope HG, Cohen BM, et al: Risk factors for neuroleptic malignant syndrome: a case control study. Arch Gen Psychiatry 46:914–918, 1989

Keck PE Jr, Seeler DC, Pope HG, et al: Porcine stress syndrome: an animal model for the neuroleptic malignant syndrome? Biol Psychiatry 28:58–62, 1990

Keck PE Jr, Pope HG, McElroy SL: Declining frequency of neuroleptic malignant syndrome in a hospital population. Am J Psychiatry 148:880–882, 1991

Keck PE Jr, Caroff SN, McElroy SL: Neuroleptic malignant syndrome and malignant hyperthermia: end of a controversy? J Neuropsychiatry Clin Neurosci 7:135–144, 1995

Kellner CH, Beale MD, Pritchett JT, et al: Electroconvulsive therapy and Parkinson's disease: the case for further study. Psychopharmacol Bull 30:495–500, 1994

Kelly D, Brull SJ: Neuroleptic malignant syndrome and mivacurium: a safe alternative to succinylcholine? Can J Anaesth 4:845–849, 1994

Keltner N, Harris CP: Serotonin syndrome: a case of fatal SSRI/MAOI interaction. Perspectives in Psychiatric Care 30:26–31, 1994

Kesavan S, Sobala GM: Serotonin syndrome with fluoxetine plus tramadol. J R Soc Med 92:474–475, 1999

Kessel JB, Verghese C, Simpson GM: Neurotoxicity related to lithium and neuroleptic combinations? A retrospective review. J Psychiatry Neurosci 17:28–30, 1992

Keyser DL, Rodnitzky RL: Neuroleptic malignant syndrome in Parkinson's disease after withdrawal or alteration of dopaminergic therapy. Arch Intern Med 151: 794–796, 1991

Khorasani A, Peruzzi WT: Dantrolene treatment for abrupt intrathecal baclofen withdrawal. Anesth Analg 80:1054–1056, 1995

Khosla R, Guntupalli KK: Heat-related illnesses. Crit Care Clin 15:251–263, 1999

Kick K: Fieberzustande unter psychopharmakotherapie: differencialtypologie und diagnostik. Pharmakopsychiatrie 14:12–20, 1981

Kilbourne EM, Choi K, Jones TS, et al: Risk factors for heatstroke: a case-control study. JAMA 247:3332–3336, 1982

Kimsey LR, Gibbs JT, Glen RS, et al: The neuroleptic malignant syndrome. Tex Med 79:54–55, 1983

Kinross-Wright VJ: Trifluoperazine and schizophrenia, in Trifluoperazine: Clinical and Pharmacologic Aspects. Edited by Brill H. Philadelphia, PA, Lea & Febiger, 1958, pp 62–70

Kirkpatrick B, Edelsohn GA: Risk factors for the neuroleptic malignant syndrome. Psychiatric Medicine 2:371–381, 1985

Kirrane R, Bodnar R, Lynch T: Response to sertraline and isocarboxazid causes a serotonin syndrome (letter). J Clin Psychopharmacol 15:144, 1995

Kish SJ, Kleinert R, Minauf M, et al: Brain neurotransmitter changes in three patients who had a fatal hyperthermia syndrome. Am J Psychiatry 147:1358–1363, 1990

Kishibayashi N, Miwa Y, Hayashi H, et al: Quinolone derivatives which may be effective in the therapy of irritable bowel syndrome. J Med Chem 36:3286–3292, 1993

Klaassen T, Ho Pian KL, Westenberg HGM, et al: Serotonin syndrome after challenge with the 5-HT agonist meta-chlorophenylpiperazine. Psychiatry Res 79:207–212, 1998

Klock JC, Boerner U, Becker EE: Coma, hyperthermia, and bleeding associated with massive LSD overdose. West J Med 120:183–188, 1973

Knochel JP: Heat stroke and related heat stress disorders. Disease-a-Month 35: 301–378, 1989

Knochel JP, Reed G: Disorders of heat regulation, in Maxwell and Kleeman's Clinical Disorders of Fluid and Electrolyte Metabolism. Edited by Narins RG. New York, McGraw-Hill, 1994, pp 1549–1590

Knoll H: [Clinical-genealogical contribution to the problem of pernicious catatonia]. Archiv fur Psychiatrie und Nervenkrantzheiten 192:1–33, 1954

Koch M, Chandragiri S, Rizvi S, et al: Catatonic signs in neuroleptic malignant syndrome. Compr Psychiatry 41:73–75, 2000

Kojima H, Terao T, Yoshimura R: Serotonin syndrome during clomipramine and lithium treatment (letter). Am J Psychiatry 150:1897, 1993

Kollias J, Bullard RW: The influence of chlorpromazine on physical and chemical mechanism of temperature regulation in the rat. J Pharmacol Exp Ther 145: 373–381, 1964

Komatsu H, Nishimura A, Okano S, et al: Neuroleptic malignant syndrome-like state in a patient with Down syndrome and basal ganglia calcification. Brain Dev 14:400–403, 1992

Konagaya M, Goto Y, Matsuoka Y: Neuroleptic malignant syndrome-like condition in multiple system atrophy. J Neurol Neurosurg Psychiatry 63:120–121, 1997

Kontaxakis V, Stefanis C, Markidis M, et al: Neuroleptic malignant syndrome in a patient with Wilson's disease (letter). J Neurol Neurosurg Psychiatry 51:1001–1002, 1988

Kopin IJ: Neurotoxins affecting biogenic aminergic neurons, in Psychopharmacology: The Third Generation of Progress. Edited by Meltzer HY. New York, Raven Press, 1987, pp 351–358

Kornhuber J, Weller M, Riederer P: Glutamate receptor antagonists for neuroleptic malignant syndrome and akinetic hyperthermic parkinsonian crisis. J Neural Transm 6:63–72, 1993

Kosten TR, Kleber HD: Sudden death in cocaine abusers: relation to neuroleptic malignant syndrome (letter). Lancet 1:1198–1199, 1987

Kosten TR, Kleber HD: Rapid death during cocaine abuse: a variant of the neuroleptic malignant syndrome? Am J Drug Alcohol Abuse 14:335–346, 1988

Kozaric-Kovacic D, Folnegovic-Smalc V, Mimica N, et al: Incidence of neuroleptic malignant syndrome during a 10-year follow-up at a psychiatric department. Neurologia Croatica 43:87–93, 1994

Koziel-Schminda E: "Ostra Smierteina Katatonia" Typu Staudera O Przebiegu Letalnym (Analiza Materialow Kliniczynch I Sekcyjnch Szpitala W Kochborowie Z Lat 1950–1970). Psychiatr Pol 7:563–567, 1973

Kraepelin E: Lectures on Clinical Psychiatry, 2nd Edition. Edited by Johnstone T. New York, William Wood, 1905

Kraines SH: Bell's mania (acute delirium). Am J Psychiatry 91:29–40, 1934

Krishna NR, Taylor MA, Abrams R: Combined haloperidol and lithium carbonate in treating manic patients. Compr Psychiatry 19:119–120, 1978

Krohn KD, Slowman-Kovacs S, Leapman SB: Cocaine and rhabdomyolysis (letter). Ann Intern Med 108:639–640, 1988

Krull F, Risse A: Neuroleptic malignant syndrome with rhabdomyolysis and therapy with physostigmine. Fortschr Neurol Psychiatr 54:398–401, 1986

Kudo K, Sasaki I, Tsuchiyama K, et al: Serotonin syndrome during clomipramine monotherapy: comparison of two diagnostic criteria. Psychiatry Clin Neurosci 51:43–46, 1997

Kuisma MJ: Fatal serotonin syndrome with trismus (letter). Ann Emerg Med 26:108, 1995

Kumagai R, Hewada T, Kurokawa K, et al: A case of impending neuroleptic malignant syndrome associated with Shy-Drager syndrome. No To Shinkei 50:745–749, 1998

Kuncl RW, Meltzer HY: Pathogenic effect of phencyclidine and restraint on rat skeletal muscle: prevention by prior denervation. Exp Neurol 45:387–402, 1974

Kuno S, Mizuta E, Yamasaki S: Neuroleptic malignant syndrome in parkinsonian patients: risk factors. Eur Neurol 38 (suppl 2):56–59, 1997

Kurlan R, Hamill R, Shoulson I: Neuroleptic malignant syndrome. Clin Neuropharmacol 7:109–120, 1984

Ladame C: Psychose aigue idiopathique ou foudroyante. Schweizer Archiv fur Neurologie und Psychiatrie 5:3–28, 1919

Lal S, Nair NPV, Guyda H: Effect of lithium on hypothalamic-pituitary dopaminergic function. Acta Psychiatr Scand 57:91–96, 1978

Lane R, Baldwin D: Selective serotonin reuptake inhibitor-induced serotonin syndrome: a review. J Clin Psychopharmacol 17:208–221, 1997

Lantz MS, Buchalter EN, Giambanco V: Serotonin syndrome following administration of tramadol with paroxetine (letter). Int J Geriatr Psychiatry 13:343–345, 1998

Lappin RI, Auchincloss EL: Treatment of the serotonin syndrome with cyproheptadine. N Engl J Med 331:1021–1022, 1994

Lauterbach EC: Catatonia-like events after valproic acid with risperidone and sertraline. Neuropsychiatry Neuropsychol Behav Neurol 11:157–163, 1998

Lazarus A: Heatstroke in a chronic schizophrenic patient treated with high-potency neuroleptics. Gen Hosp Psychiatry 7:361–363, 1985a

Lazarus A: Neuroleptic malignant syndrome and amantadine withdrawal (letter). Am J Psychiatry 142:142, 1985b

Lazarus A: Neuroleptic malignant syndrome: detection and management. Psychiatric Annals 15:706–712, 1985c

Lazarus A, Rosenberg H: Malignant hyperthermia during ECT. Am J Psychiatry 148:541–542, 1991

Lazarus AL, Toglia JU: Fatal myoglobinuric renal failure in a patient with tardive dyskinesia. Neurology 35:1055–1057, 1985

Lazarus A, Mann SC, Caroff SN: The Neuroleptic Malignant Syndrome and Related Conditions. Washington, DC, American Psychiatric Press, 1989

Lazarus AL, Morre KE, Spinner NB: Recurrent neuroleptic malignant syndrome associated with inv dup (15) and mental retardation. Clin Genet 39:65–67, 1991

Lee JWY: Serum iron in catatonia and neuroleptic malignant syndrome. Biol Psychiatry 44:499–507, 1998

Lee JWY: Catatonic and non-catatonic neuroleptic malignant syndrome (letter). Aust N Z J Psychiatry 34:877, 2000

Lee JWY, Robertson S: Clozapine withdrawal catatonia and neuroleptic malignant syndrome: a case report. Ann Clin Psychiatry 9:165–169, 1997

Lee S, Merriam A, Kim TS, et al: Cerebellar degeneration in neuroleptic malignant syndrome: neuropathologic findings and review of the literature concerning heat-related nervous system injury. J Neurol Neurosurg Psychiatry 52:387–391, 1989

Lee TF, Mora F, Myers RD: Dopamine and thermoregulation: an evaluation with special reference to dopaminergic pathways. Neurosci Biobehav Rev 9:589–598, 1985

Lees H: The effects of 1-(1-phenyl cyclohexl) piperidine hydrochloride (sernyl) on rat liver mitochondria. Neuropharmacol 20:306, 1961

Lefkowitz D, Ford CS, Rich C, et al: Cerebellar syndrome following neuroleptic induced heatstroke. J Neurol Neurosurg Psychiatry 46:183–185, 1983

Lejoyeux M, Fineyre F, Ades J: The serotonin syndrome (letter). Am J Psychiatry 149:1410–1411, 1992

Lejoyeux M, Rouillon F, Ades J: Prospective evaluation of the serotonin syndrome in depressed inpatients treated with clomipramine. Acta Psychiatr Scand 88: 369–371, 1993

Lenzi A, Raffaelli S, Marazziti D: Serotonin syndrome-like symptoms in a patient with obsessive-compulsive disorder, following inappropriate increase in fluvoxamine dosage. Pharmacopsychiatry 26:100–101, 1993

Lesaca T: Amoxapine and neuroleptic malignant syndrome (letter). Am J Psychiatry 144:1514, 1987

Levenson JL: Neuroleptic malignant syndrome. Am J Psychiatry 142:1137–1145, 1985

Levenson JL: Clinical differentiation between lethal catatonia and neuroleptic malignant syndrome (letter). Am J Psychiatry 146:1240–1241, 1989

Levinson DF, Simpson GM: Neuroleptic-induced extrapyramidal symptoms with fever: heterogeneity of the "neuroleptic malignant syndrome." Arch Gen Psychiatry 43:839–848, 1986

Lieberman A, Gopinathan G: Treatment of "on-off" phenomena with lithium (letter). Ann Neurol 12:402, 1982

Lin MT: Effects of dopaminergic antagonists and agonists on thermoregulation in rabbits. J Physiol 293:217–228, 1979

Lin MT, Wang HC, Chandra A: The effects on thermoregulation of intracerebroventricular injection of acetylcholine, pilocarpine, physostigmine, atropine and hemicholinium in the rat. Neuropharmacology 18:561–565, 1980

Lin MT, Tsay HJ, Su WH, et al: Changes in extracellular serotonin in rat hypothalamus affect thermoregulatory function. Am J Physiol 274 (5, pt 2):R1260–R1267, 1998

Lingjaerde O: Contributions to the study of schizophrenia and the acute, malignant deliria. Journal of the Oslo City Hospital 14:43–83, 1963

Linnoila M, Karoum F, Rosenthal N, et al: Electroconvulsive treatment and lithium carbonate: their effects on norepinephrine metabolism in patients with primary major depressions. Arch Gen Psychiatry 40:677–680, 1983

Litovitz TL, Troutman WG: Amoxapine overdose: seizures and fatalities. JAMA 250:1069–1071, 1983

Logan AC, Stickle B, O'Keefe N, et al: Survival following "ecstasy" ingestion with a peak temperature of 42 degree Celsius. Anaesthesia 48:1017–1018, 1993

Loghmanee F, Tobak M: Fatal malignant hyperthermia associated with recreational cocaine and ethanol abuse. Am J Forensic Med Pathol 7:246–248, 1986

Lohr JB, Wisenewski AA: Catatonia, in The Neuropsychiatric Basis of Movement Disorders. Edited by Lohr JB, Wisenewski AA. Baltimore, MD, Guilford, 1987, pp 201–247

Lomax P, Schonbaum E: The effects of drugs on thermoregulation during exposure to hot environments. Prog Brain Res 115:193–204, 1998

Lou J-S: Pathophysiology of basal ganglia disorders. CNS Spectrums 3:36–40, 1998

Louilot A, Le Moal M, Simon H: Opposite influences of dopaminergic pathways to the prefrontal cortex or the septum on the dopaminergic transmission in the nucleus accumbens: an in vivo voltammetric study. Neuroscience 29:45–56, 1989

Lowance D: Heat injury: a possible association with lithium carbonate therapy. J Med Assoc Ga 69:284–286, 1980

Lu CS, Ryu SJ: Neuroleptic malignant-like syndrome associated with acute hydrocephalus. Mov Disord 6:381–383, 1991

Lutz EG: Neuroleptic-induced akathisia and dystonia triggered by alcohol. JAMA 236:2422–2423, 1976

MacKay FJ, Dunn NR, Mann RD: Antidepressants and the serotonin syndrome in general practice. Br J Gen Pract 49:871–874, 1999

Maggi A, Enna SJ: Regional alterations in rat brain neurotransmitter systems following chronic lithium treatment. J Neurochem 34:888–892, 1980

Malamud N, Haymaker W, Custer RP: Heatstroke: a clinico-pathologic study of 125 fatal cases. Military Surgeon 99:397–449, 1946

Maling TJB, MacDonald AD, Davis M, et al: Neuroleptic malignant syndrome: a review of the Wellington experience. N Z Med J 101:193–195, 1988

Mandac BR, Harvitz EA, Nelson VS: Hyperthermia associated with baclofen withdrawal and increased spasticity. Arch Phys Med Rehabil 74:96–97, 1993

Mann SC, Boger WP: Psychotropic drugs, summer heat and humidity, and hyperpyrexia: a danger restated. Am J Psychiatry 135:1097–1100, 1978

Mann SC, Caroff SN: Lethal catatonia and the neuroleptic malignant syndrome, in Psychiatry: A World Perspective, Vol 3. Edited by Stefanis CN, Rabavilas AD, Soldatos CR. Amsterdam, Elsevier Science, 1990, pp 287–292

Mann SC, Greenstein RA, Eilers R: Early onset of severe dyskinesia following lithium-haloperidol treatment. Am J Psychiatry 140:1385–1386, 1983

Mann SC, Caroff SN, Bleier HR, et al: Lethal catatonia. Am J Psychiatry 143:1374–1381, 1986

Mann SC, Caroff SN, Bleier HR, et al: Electroconvulsive therapy of the lethal catatonia syndrome: case report and review. Convulsive Therapy 6:239–247, 1990

Mann SC, Caroff SN, Lazarus A: Pathogenesis of neuroleptic malignant syndrome. Psychiatric Annals 21:175–180, 1991

Mann SC, Gliatto MF, Campbell EC, et al: Psychotic disorders, in Psychiatry for Primary Care Providers. Edited by Gliatto MF, Caroff SN, Kaiser R. Washington, DC, American Psychiatric Press, 1999, pp 107–133

Mann SC, Caroff SN, Fricchione G, et al: Central dopamine hypoactivity and the pathogenesis of the neuroleptic malignant syndrome. Psychiatric Annals 30: 363–374, 2000

Mann SC, Auriacombe M, Macfadden W, et al: [Lethal catatonia: clinical aspects and therapeutic intervention. A review of the literature]. Encephale 27:213–216, 2001

Mann SC, Caroff SN, Campbell, et al: The malignant catatonia syndrome. Paper presented at the 155th annual meeting of the American Psychiatric Association, Philadelphia, PA, May 18–23, 2002

Mann SC, Caroff SN, Fricchione G, et al: Malignant catatonia, in Catatonia: From Psychopathology to Neurobiology. Edited by Caroff SN, Mann SC, Francis A, et al. Washington, DC, American Psychiatric Publishing (in press)

Manor I, Hermesh H, Munitz H, et al: Neuroleptic malignant syndrome with gangliosidosis type II. Biol Psychiatry 41:1222–1224, 1997

Manor I, Hermesh H, Valaevski A, et al: Recurrence pattern of serum creatine phosphokinase levels in repeated acute psychosis. Biol Psychiatry 43:288–292, 1998

Margolese HC, Chouinard G: Serotonin syndrome from addition of low-dose trazodone to nefazodone (letter). Am J Psychiatry 157:1022, 2000

Martin ML, Lucid EJ, Walker RW: Neuroleptic malignant syndrome. Ann Emerg Med 14:354–358, 1985

Marzuk PM, Tarditt K, Leon AC, et al: Ambient temperature and mortality from unintentional cocaine overdose. JAMA 279:1795–1800, 1998

Mason BJ, Blackburn KH: Possible serotonin syndrome associated with tramadol and sertraline coadministration. Ann Pharmacother 31:175–177, 1997

Mason PJ, Morris VA, Balcezak TJ: Serotonin syndrome: presentation of 2 cases and review of the literature. Medicine (Baltimore) 79:201–209, 2000

Mathew NT, Tietjen GE, Lucker C: Serotonin syndrome complicating migraine pharmacotherapy. Cephalgia 16:323–327, 1996

May DC, Morris SW, Stewart RM, et al: Neuroleptic malignant syndrome: response to dantrolene sodium. Ann Intern Med 98:183–184, 1983

McCarron MM, Schulze BW, Thompson GA, et al: Acute phencyclidine intoxication: clinical patterns, complications, and treatment. Ann Emerg Med 10:290–297, 1981a

McCarron MM, Schulze BW, Thompson GA, et al: Acute phencyclidine intoxication: incidence of clinical findings in 1000 cases. Ann Emerg Med 10:237–242, 1981b

McGugan EA: Hyperpyrexia in the emergency department. Emergency Medicine (Fremantle) 13:116–120, 2001

McKenna DJ, Peroutka SJ: Neurochemistry and neurotoxicity of 3,4-methylenedioxy methamphetamine (MDMA, "Ecstasy"). J Neurochem 54:14–22, 1990

Meador-Woodruff JH, Damask SP, Wang J, et al: Dopamine receptor mRNA expression in human striatum and neocortex. Neuropsychopharmacology 15:17–29, 1996

Mega MS, Cummings JL: Frontal-subcortical circuits and neuropsychiatric disorders. J Neuropsychiatry Clin Neurosci 6:358–370, 1994

Mega MS, Cummings JL, Salloway S, et al: The limbic system: an anatomic, phylogenetic, and clinical perspective, in The Neuropsychiatry of Limbic and Subcortical Disorders. Edited by Salloway S, Malloy P, Cummings JL. Washington, DC, American Psychiatric Press, 1997, pp 3–18

Mekler G, Woggon B: A case of serotonin syndrome caused by venlafaxine and lithium. Pharmacopsychiatry 30:272–273, 1997

Meller E, Friedman E: Lithium dissociates haloperidol-induced behavioral super-sensitivity from reduced DOPAC increase in rat striatum. Eur J Pharmacol 76: 25–29, 1981

Meltzer HY: Rigidity, hyperpyrexia and coma following fluphenazine enanthate. Psychopharmacologia 29:337–346, 1973

Meltzer HY: Treatment of the neuroleptic-nonresponsive schizophrenic patient. Schizophr Bull 18:515–542, 1992

Meltzer HY: The role of serotonin in antipsychotic drug action. Neuropsychophar-macology 21:106S–115S, 1999

Meltzer HY, Holtzman PS, Hassu SJ, et al: Effect of phencyclidine and stress on plasma creatine phosphokinase (CPK) and aldolase activity in man. Psycho-pharmacologia 26:44–53, 1972

Meltzer HY, Matsubara S, Lee JC: Classification of typical and atypical antipsy-chotics on the basis of dopamine D1, D2 and serotonin2 pKi values. J Pharma-col Exp Ther 251:238–246, 1989

Meltzer HY, Cola PA, Parsa M: Marked elevations of serum creatine kinase activity associated with antipsychotic drug treatment. Neuropsychopharmacology 15: 395–405, 1996

Merigian KS, Roberts JR: Cocaine intoxication: hyperpyrexia, rhabdomyolysis and acute renal failure. Clinical Toxicology 25:135–148, 1987

Merriam AE: Neuroleptic malignant syndrome after imipramine withdrawal (let-ter). J Clin Psychopharmacol 7:53–54, 1987

Millan MJ: Improving the treatment of schizophrenia: focus on serotonin (5-HT) 1A receptors. J Pharmacol Exp Ther 295:853–861, 2000

Millan MJ, Audinot V, Rivet J-C, et al: S 14297, a novel selective ligand at cloned human D-3 receptors, blocks 7-OH-DPAT-induced hypothermia in rats. Eur J Pharmacol 260:R3–R5, 1994

Millan MJ, Peglion JL, Vian J, et al: Functional correlates of dopamine D3 receptor activation in the rat in vivo and their modulation by the selective antagonist, (+)–S 14297, 1: activation of postsynaptic D3 receptors mediates hypothermia, whereas blockade of D2 receptors elicits prolactin secretion and catalepsy. J Pharmacol Exp Ther 275:885–898, 1995

Millan MJ, Gobert A, Newman-Tancredi A, et al: S 16924 ((R)-2-[1-[2-(2,3-dihy-dro-benzo [1,4] dioxin-5-Yloxy)-ethyl]-pyrrolidin-3yl]-1-(4-fluoro-phenyl)-ethanone), a novel, potential antipsychotic with marked serotonin (5-HT) 1A agonist properties, I: receptorial and neurochemical profile in comparison with clozapine and haloperidol. J Pharmacol Exp Ther 286:1341–1355, 1998

Miller F, Menninger J: Correlation of neuroleptic dose and neurotoxicity in pa-tients given lithium and a neuroleptic. Hospital and Community Psychiatry 38:1219–1221, 1987a

Miller F, Menninger J: Lithium-neuroleptic neurotoxicity is dose dependent. J Clin Psychopharmacol 7:89–91, 1987b

Miller F, Friedman R, Tanenbaum J, et al: Disseminated intravascular coagulation and acute myoglobinuric renal failure: a consequence of the serotonergic syn-drome (letter). J Clin Psychopharmacol 11:277–278, 1991

Mills KC: Serotonin syndrome: a clinical update. Crit Care Clin 13:763–783, 1997

Mitchell RS: Fatal toxic encephalitis occurring during iproniazid therapy in pulmonary tuberculosis. Ann Intern Med 42:417–424, 1955

Miyaoka H, Kamijima K: Encephalopathy during amitriptyline therapy: are neuroleptic malignant syndrome and serotonin syndrome spectrum disorders (letter)? Int Clin Psychopharmacol 10:265–267, 1995

Miyaoka H, Shishikura K, Otsubo T, et al: Diazepam-responsive neuroleptic malignant syndrome: a diagnostic subtype? Am J Psychiatry 154:882, 1997

Miyatake R, Iwahashi K, Matsushita M, et al: No association between the neuroleptic malignant syndrome and mutations in the RYR1 gene associated with malignant hyperthermia. J Neurol Sci 143:161–165, 1996

Modestin J, Toffler G, Dresher JP: Neuroleptic malignant syndrome: results of a prospective study. Psychiatry Res 44:251–256, 1992

Molaie M: Serotonin syndrome presenting with migraine-like stroke. Headache 37: 519–521, 1997

Morris HH, McCormick WF, Reinarz JA: Neuroleptic malignant syndrome. Arch Neurol 37:462–463, 1980

Moyes DG: Malignant hyperpyrexia caused by trimeprazine. Br J Anaesth 45:1163–1164, 1973

Mueller PD, Korey WS: Death by "ecstasy": the serotonin syndrome? Ann Emerg Med 32:377–380, 1998

Mueller PS: Neuroleptic malignant syndrome. Psychosomatics 26:654–662, 1985

Mueller PS, Vester JW, Fermaglich J: Neuroleptic malignant syndrome: successful treatment with bromocriptine. JAMA 249:386–388, 1983

Muly EC, McDonald W, Steffens D, et al: Serotonin syndrome produced by a combination of fluoxetine and lithium (letter). Am J Psychiatry 150:1565, 1993

Murthy VS, Wilkes RG, Roberts NB: Creatine kinase isoform changes following ecstasy overdose. Anaesth Intensive Care 25:156–159, 1997

Naganuma H, Fujii I: Incidence and risk factors in neuroleptic malignant syndrome. Acta Psychiatr Scand 90:424–426, 1994

National Center for Health Statistics: Compressed Mortality File. Atlanta, GA, U.S. Department of Health and Human Services, Centers for Disease Control and Prevention, 2000

Neil JF, Himmelhoch JM, Licata SM: Emergence of myasthenia gravis during treatment with lithium carbonate. Arch Gen Psychiatry 33:1090–1092, 1976

Nemes ZC, Volavka J, Lajtha A, et al: Concurrent lithium administration results in higher haloperidol levels in brain and plasma of guinea pigs. Psychiatry Res 20: 313–316, 1987

Neumarker KJ, Dudeck U, Plaza P: Borrelicn-enzephalitis und katatonie im jugendalter. Nervenarzt 60:115–119, 1989

Neuvonen PJ, Pohjola-Sintonen S, Tacke U, et al: Five fatal cases of serotonin syndrome after moclobemide-citalopram overdoses (letter). Lancet 342:1419, 1993

Newman PK, Saunders M: Lithium neurotoxicity. Postgrad Med J 55:701–703, 1979

Nicklason FN, Finuccine PM, Pathy MSJ: Neuroleptic malignant syndrome—an unrecognized problem in elderly patients with psychiatric illness? Int J Geriatr Psychiatry 6:171–175, 1991

Nierenberg DW, Semprebon M: The central nervous system serotonin syndrome. Clin Pharmacol Ther 53:84–88, 1993

Nimmagadda SR, Ryan DH, Atkin SL: Neuroleptic malignant syndrome after venlafaxine. Lancet 354:289–290, 2000

Nimmo SM, Kennedy BW, Tullett WM, et al: Drug-induced hyperthermia. Anaesthesia 48:892–895, 1993

Ninan I, Kulkarni SK: Partial agonist action of clozapine at dopamine D-2 receptors in dopamine depleted animals. Psychopharmacology 135:311–317, 1998

Ninan I, Kulkarni SK: Antagonism by pimozide of olanzapine-induced hypothermia. Fundam Clin Pharmacol 13:541–546, 1999a

Ninan I, Kulkarni SK: Differential effects of olanzapine at dopamine D1 and D2 receptors in dopamine depleted animals. Psychopharmacology (Berl) 142:175–181, 1999b

Nisijima K: Abnormal monoamine metabolism in cerebrospinal fluid in a case of serotonin syndrome. J Clin Psychopharmacol 20:107–108, 2000

Nisijima K, Ishiguro T: Neuroleptic malignant syndrome: a study of CSF monoamine metabolism. Biol Psychiatry 27:280–288, 1990

Nisijima K, Ishiguro T: Cerebrospinal fluid levels of monoamine metabolites and gamma-aminobutyric acid in neuroleptic malignant syndrome. J Psychiatr Res 29:233–244, 1995a

Nisijima K, Ishiguro T: Does dantrolene influence central dopamine and serotonin metabolism in the neuroleptic malignant syndrome? A retrospective study. Biol Psychiatry 33:45–48, 1995b

Nisijima K, Ishiguro T: Electroconvulsive therapy for the treatment of neuroleptic malignant syndrome with psychotic symptoms: a report of five cases. J ECT 15:158–163, 1999

Nisijima K, Shimizu M, Abe T, et al: A case of serotonin syndrome induced by concomitant treatment with low-dose trazodone and amitriptyline and lithium. Int Clin Psychopharmacol 11:289–290, 1996

Nisijima K, Noguti M, Ishiguro T: Intravenous injection of levodopa is more effective than dantrolene as therapy for neuroleptic malignant syndrome. Biol Psychiatry 41:913–914, 1997

Nisijima K, Yoshino T, Yui K, et al: Potent serotonin (5-HT)(2A) receptor antagonists completely prevent the development of hyperthermia in an animal model of the 5-HT syndrome. Brain Res 890:23–31, 2001

Nitenson NC, Kando JC, Frankenburg FR, et al: Fever associated with clozapine administration (letter). Am J Psychiatry 152:1102, 1995

Nolen WA, Zwann WA: Treatment of lethal catatonia with electroconvulsive therapy and dantrolene sodium: a case report. Acta Psychiatr Scand 82:90–92, 1990

Norman AB, Wylie GL, Prince AK: Supersensitivity of d-amphetamine-induced hyperthermia in rats following continuous treatment with neuroleptics. Eur J Pharmacol 140:349–351, 1987

Noyer CM, Schwartz BM: Sertraline, a selective serotonin reuptake inhibitor, unmasking carcinoid syndrome. Am Gastroenterol 92:1387–1388, 1997

Nunes JL, Sharif NA, Michel AD, et al: Dopamine D2 receptors mediate hypothermia in mice: icv and ip effects of agonists and antagonists. Neurochem Res 16:1167–1174, 1991

Oates JA, Sjoerdsma A: Neurologic effects of tryptophan in patients receiving a monoamine oxidase inhibitor. Neurology 10:1076–1078, 1960

Oerther S, Ahlenius S: Atypical antipsychotics and dopamine D1 receptor agonism: an in vitro experimental study using core temperature measurements in the rat. J Pharmacol Exp Ther 292:731–736, 2000

Ohman R, Spigset O: Serotonin syndrome induced by fluvoxamine-lithium interaction (letter). Pharmacopsychiatry 26:263–264, 1993

Olson KR, Benowitz NL: Life-threatening cocaine intoxication. Problems in Critical Care 1:95–105, 1987

Ooi TK: The serotonin syndrome (letter). BMJ 308:456, 1995

Orland RM, Daghestani AN: A case of catatonia induced by bacterial meningoencephalitis. J Clin Psychiatry 48:489–490, 1987

Ostrow DG, Sontham AS, Davis JM: Lithium-drug interactions altering the intracellular lithium level: an in-vitro study. Biol Psychiatry 15:723–739, 1980

Otani K, Hariuchi M, Kondo T, et al: Is the predisposition to neuroleptic malignant syndrome genetically transmitted? Br J Psychiatry 158:850–853, 1991

Page P, Morgan M, Loh L: Ketamine anesthesia in pediatric procedures. Acta Anaesthesiol Scand 16:155–160, 1972

Pandey GN, Goel I, Davis JM: Effect of neuroleptic drugs on lithium uptake for the human erythrocyte. Clin Pharmacol Ther 26:96–102, 1979

Pao M, Tipnis T: Serotonin syndrome after sertraline overdose in a 5-year-old girl. Arch Pediatr Adolesc Med 151:1064–1067, 1997

Parada MA, Parada MP, Rada D, et al: Sulpiride increases and dopamine decreases intracranial temperature in rats when injected in the lateral hypothalamus: an animal model for the neuroleptic malignant syndrome? Brain Res 674:117–121, 1995

Pare CMB, Sandler M: A clinical and biochemical study of a trial of iproniazid in the treatment of depression. J Neurol Neurosurg Psychiatry 22:247–251, 1959

Parris C, Mack JM, Cochiolo JA, et al: Hypothermia in 2 patients treated with atypical antipsychotic medication (letter). J Clin Psychiatry 62:61–63, 2001

Patel P, Bristow G: Postoperative neuroleptic malignant syndrome: a case report. Can J Anaesth 34:515–518, 1987

Pearlman CA Jr: Neuroleptic malignant syndrome: a review of the literature. J Clin Psychopharmacol 6:257–273, 1986

Pearlman CA Jr: NMS and catatonia: one syndrome or two? Paper presented at the 153rd annual meeting of the American Psychiatric Association, Chicago, IL, May 13–18, 2000

Pennati A, Sacchetti E, Calzeroni A: Dantrolene in lethal catatonia (letter). Am J Psychiatry 148:268, 1991

Perachon S, Betancur C, Pilon C, et al: Role of dopamine D-3 receptors in thermoregulation: a reappraisal. Neuroreport 11:221–225, 2000

Perera KMH, Ferraro A, Pinto MRM: Catatonia LSD induced? Aust N Z J Psychiatry 29:324–327, 1995

Perry N: Venlafaxine-induced serotonin syndrome with relapse following amitriptyline. Postgrad Med J 76:254–256, 2000

Pert A, Rosenblatt JE, Sivit C, et al: Long term treatment with lithium prevents the development of dopamine receptor supersensitivity. Science 201:171–173, 1978

Pestronk A, Drachman DB: Lithium reduces the number of acetylcholine receptors in skeletal muscle. Science 210:342–343, 1980

Pfeiffer RF, Sucha EL: On-off induced malignant hyperthermia. Ann Neurol 18: 138–139, 1985

Phan TG, Yu RY, Hersch MI: Hypothermia induced by risperidone and olanzapine in a patient with Prader-Willi syndrome (letter). Med J Aust 169:230–231, 1998

Philbrick KL, Rummans TA: Malignant catatonia. J Neuropsychiatry Clin Neurosci 6:1–13, 1994

Phillips S, Ringo P: Phenelzine and venlafaxine interaction. Am J Psychiatry 152: 1400–1401, 1995

Physicians' Desk Reference, 56th Edition. Montvale, NJ, Medical Economics, 2002

Pittman KJ, Jakubavic A, Febiger HC: The effects of chronic lithium on behavioral and biochemical indices of dopamine receptor supersensitivity in the rat. Psychopharmacology 82:371–377, 1984

Pollmacher T, Hinze-Selch D, Fenzel T, et al: Plasma levels of cytokine receptors during treatment with haloperidol. Am J Psychiatry 154:1763–1765, 1997

Pollmacher T, Haack M, Schuld A, et al: Effects of antipsychotic drugs on cytokine networks. J Psychiatr Res 34:369–382, 2000

Pollock N, Hodges M, Sendell J: Prolonged malignant hyperthermia in the absence of triggering agents. Anaesth Intensive Care 20:520–523, 1992

Pollock N, Hodges M, Sendell J: Reply to neuroleptic malignant syndrome and malignant hyperthermia (letter). Anaesth Intensive Care 21:478–479, 1993

Pope HG Jr, Keck PE Jr, McElroy SL: Frequency and presentation of neuroleptic malignant syndrome in a large psychiatric hospital. Am J Psychiatry 143:1227–1233, 1986

Pope HG, Aizley HG, Keck PE, et al: Neuroleptic malignant syndrome: long-term follow-up of 20 cases. J Clin Psychiatry 52:208–212, 1991

Portfl L, Hilbert D, Gruson JC, et al: Malignant hyperthermia and neuroleptic malignant syndrome in a patient during treatment for acute asthma. Acta Anesthesiol Scand 43:107–110, 1999

Power BM, Pinder M, Hackett LP, et al: Fatal serotonin syndrome following a combined overdose of moclobemide, clomipramine and fluoxetine. Anaesth Intensive Care 23:499–502, 1995

Powers P, Douglass TS, Waziri R: Hyperpyrexia in catatonic states. Diseases of the Nervous System 37:359–361, 1976

Prabhakar S, Malhotra RM, Goel DS: Rabies presenting as catatonic stupor. J Assoc Physicians India 40:272–273, 1992

Prakash R, Kelwala S, Ban TA: Neurotoxicity with combined administration of lithium and a neuroleptic. Compr Psychiatry 23:567–571, 1982

Price LH, Charney DS, Heninger GR: Serotonin syndrome. Am J Psychiatry 149: 1116–1117, 1992

Primeau F, Fontaine R, Chouinard G: Poorly controlled EPS: risk factors for NMS. Can J Psychiatry 32:238–329, 1987

Przewlocka B, Kaluza J: The effect of intraventricularly administered noradrenaline and dopamine on the body temperature of the rat. Polish Journal of Pharmacology and Pharmacy 25:345–355, 1973

Pumariega AJ, Muller B, Rivers-Bulkeley N: Acute renal failure secondary to amoxapine overdose. JAMA 248:3141–3142, 1982

Pycock CL, Kerwin RW, Carter CJ: Effects of lesion of cortical dopamine terminals on subcortical dopamine receptors in rats. Nature 286:74–76, 1980

Quinn NP: Levodopa, in Handbook of Parkinson's Disease. Edited by Koller WC. New York, Marcel Dekker, 1987, pp 317–337

Rainer C, Scheinost NA, Lefeber EJ: Neuroleptic malignant syndrome: when levodopa withdrawal is the cause. Postgrad Med 89:175–178, 1991

Ram A, Cao Q, Keck PE Jr, et al: Structural change in dopamine D_2 receptor gene in a patient with neuroleptic malignant syndrome. Am J Med Genet 60:228–230, 1995

Rao R: Serotonin syndrome associated with trazodone (letter). Int J Geriatr Psychiatry 12:129–130, 1997

Rao TS, Kim HS, Lehmann J, et al: Differential effects of phencyclidine (PCP) and ketamine on mesocortical and mesostriatal dopamine release in vivo. Life Sci 45:1065–1072, 1989

Rappolt RJ, Gay GR, Farris RD: Emergency management of acute phencyclidine intoxication. Journal of the American College of Emergency Physicians 8:68–76, 1979

Rascol O, Salachas F, Montastruc JL: [Neuroleptic malignant-like syndrome following levodopa withdrawal]. Rev Neurol (Paris) 146:215–218, 1990

Rasmussen H: The calcium messenger system I. N Engl J Med 314:1094–1100, 1986a

Rasmussen H: The calcium messenger system II. N Engl J Med 314:1164–1170, 1986b

Ravi SD, Borge GF, Roach FL, et al: Neuroleptics, laryngeal-pharyngeal dystonia, and acute renal failure (letter). J Clin Psychiatry 43:300, 1982

Reches A, Fahn S: Lithium in the "on-off" phenomenon. Ann Neurol 14:91–92, 1983

Reches A, Wagner HR, Jackson V, et al: Chronic lithium administration has no effect on haloperidol induced supersensitivity of pre- and postsynaptic dopamine receptors in rat brain. Brain Res 246:172–177, 1982

Reches A, Jackson-Lewis V, Fahn S: Lithium does not interact with haloperidol in the dopaminergic pathways of the rat brain. Psychopharmacology 82:330–334, 1984

Reda FA, Escobar JI, Scanlow JM: Lithium carbonate in the treatment of tardive dyskinesia. Am J Psychiatry 132:560–562, 1975

Reeves RK, Stolp-Smith KA, Christopherson MV: Hyperthermia, rhabdomyolysis, and disseminated intravascular coagulation associated with baclofen pump catheter failure. Arch Phys Med Rehabil 79:353–356, 1998

Reeves RR, Bullen JA: Serotonin syndrome produced by paroxetine and low-dose trazodone (letter). Psychosomatics 36:159–160, 1995

Rella JG, Hoffman RS: Possible serotonin syndrome from paroxetine and clonazepam (letter). Clin Toxicol 36:257–258, 1998

Renfordt E, Wardin B: Elektrokrampf-und dantrolen behandlung einer akuten febrilen katatonie. Nervenarzt 56:153–156, 1985

Renshaw PF, Joseph NE, Leigh JS: Chronic dietary lithium induces increased levels of myo-inositol-1-phosphatase activity in rat cerebral cortex homogenates. Brain Res 380:401–404, 1986a

Renshaw PF, Summers JJ, Renshaw CE, et al: Changes in the ^{31}P-NMR spectra of cats receiving lithium chloride systemically. Biol Psychiatry 21:694–698, 1986b

Renyi L: The involvement of the 5-HT$_1$ and 5-HT$_2$ receptors and of catecholaminergic systems in different components of the 5-HT syndrome in the rat. Polish Journal of Pharmacology and Pharmacy 43:405–419, 1991

Ricaurte GA, De Lanney LE, Irwin I, et al: Toxic effects of MDMA on central serotonergic neurons in the primate: importance of route and frequency of drug administration. Brain Res 446:165–168, 1988

Richard I, Kurlan R, Tanner C, et al: Serotonin syndrome and the combined use of Deprenyl and an antidepressant in Parkinson's disease. Neurology 48:1070–1077, 1997

Rifkin A, Quitkin F, Klein DF: Organic brain syndrome during lithium carbonate therapy. Compr Psychiatry 14:251–254, 1973

Ritchie P: Neuroleptic malignant syndrome. BMJ 287:560–561, 1983

Rivera-Calimlin L, Kerzner B, Karch FE: Effect of lithium on plasma chlorpromazine levels. Clin Pharmacol Ther 23:451–455, 1978

Roberts AN: The value of ECT in delirium. Br J Psychiatry 109:653–655, 1963

Roberts JR, Quattrocchi E, Howland MA: Severe hyperthermia secondary to intravenous drug abuse (letter). Am J Emerg Med 2:373, 1984

Roberts L, Wright H: Survival following intentional massive overdose of 'Ecstasy.' J Accid Emerg Med 11:53–54, 1994

Roervik S, Stovner J: Ketamine-induced acidosis, fever and creatine kinase rise. Lancet 2:1384–1385, 1974

Rogers JD, Stoudemire GA: Neuroleptic malignant syndrome in multiple sclerosis: possible masking effects of antispasmodics. Psychosomatics 29:221–223, 1988

Rosebush PI, Mazurek MF: Serum iron and neuroleptic malignant syndrome. Lancet 338:149–151, 1991

Rosebush PI, Stewart T: A prospective analysis of 24 episodes of neuroleptic malignant syndrome. Am J Psychiatry 146:717–725, 1989

Rosebush PI, Stewart TD, Gelenberg AJ: Twenty neuroleptic rechallenges after neuroleptic malignant syndrome in 15 patients. J Clin Psychiatry 50:295–298, 1989

Rosebush PI, Stewart T, Mazurek MF: The treatment of neuroleptic malignant syndrome: are dantrolene and bromocriptine useful adjuncts to supportive care? Br J Psychiatry 159:709–712, 1991

Rosebush PI, Margetts P, Mazurek MF: Serotonin syndrome as a result of clomipramine monotherapy. J Clin Psychopharmacol 19:285–287, 1999

Rosenbaum JF, Fava M, Hoog SL, et al: Selective serotonin reuptake inhibitor discontinuation syndrome: a randomized clinical trial. Biol Psychiatry 44:77–87, 1998

Rosenberg H, Fletcher JE: An update on the malignant hyperthermia syndrome. Ann Acad Med Singapore 23 (suppl):84–97, 1994

Rosenberg MR, Green M: Neuroleptic malignant syndrome: review of response to therapy. Arch Intern Med 149:1927–1931, 1989

Rosenblatt JE, Pert A, Layton B, et al: Chronic lithium reduces [^{3}H]-spiroperidol binding in rat striatum. Eur J Pharmacol 67:321–322, 1980

Ross-Canada J, Chizzonite RA, Meltzer HY: Retention of sarcoplasmic calcium inhibits development of the phencyclidine-restraint experimental myopathy. Exp Neurol 79:1–10, 1983

Rosse R, Ciolino C: Dopamine agonists and neuroleptic malignant syndrome. Am J Psychiatry 142:270–271, 1985

Roth B, Buckley PE, Schulz SC: Molecular biology and antipsychotic medications, in Schizophrenia in a Molecular Age. Edited by Tamminga CA (Review of Psychiatry Series; Oldham JM and Riba MB, series eds.). Washington, DC, American Psychiatric Press, 1999, pp 141–168

Roth D, Alarcon FJ, Fernandez JA, et al: Acute rhabdomyolysis associated with cocaine intoxication. N Engl J Med 319:673–677, 1988

Roth SD, Addonizio G, Susman VL: Diagnosing and treating neuroleptic malignant syndrome (letter). Am J Psychiatry 143:673, 1986

Rothke S, Bush D: Neuropsychological sequelae of neuroleptic malignant syndrome. Biol Psychiatry 21:838–841, 1986

Roxanas MG, Machado F: Serotonin syndrome in combined moclobemide and venlafaxine ingestion (letter). Med J Aust 168:523–524, 1998

Rubin RL: Adolescent infectious mononucleosis with psychosis. J Clin Psychiatry 39:773–775, 1978

Rubio-Gozalbo ME, van Waardenburg DA, Forget PP, et al: Neuroleptic malignant syndrome during zuclopenthixol therapy in X-linked cerebral adrenoleukodystrophy. J Inherit Metab Dis 24:605–606, 2001

Rudnick G, Wall SC: The molecular mechanism of "ecstasy" [3,4-methylene dioxymethamphetamine (MDMA)]: serotonin transporters are targets for MDMA-induced serotonin release. Proc Natl Acad Sci U S A 89:1817–1821, 1992

Rummans TA: NMS as malignant catatonia. Paper presented at the 153rd annual meeting of the American Psychiatric Association, Chicago, IL, May 13–18, 2000

Ruwe WD, Myers RD: Dopamine in the hypothalamus of the cat: pharmacological characterization and push-pull perfusion analysis of sites mediating hypothermia. Pharmacol Biochem Behav 9:65–80, 1978

Sachdev PS: Lithium potentiation of neuroleptic-related extrapyramidal side effects (letter). Am J Psychiatry 143:942, 1986

Sachdev P, Kruk J, Kneebone M, et al: Clozapine-induced neuroleptic malignant syndrome: review and report of new cases. J Clin Psychopharmacol 15:365–371, 1995

Sachdev P, Mason C, Hadzi-Pavlovic D: Case-control study of neuroleptic malignant syndrome. Am J Psychiatry 154:1156–1158, 1997

Sakkas P, Davis JM, Hua J, et al: Pharmacotherapy of neuroleptic malignant syndrome. Psychiatric Annals 21:157–164, 1991

Salmi P: Independent roles of dopamine D-1 and D-2/3 receptors in rat thermoregulation. Brain Res 781:188–193, 1998

Salmi P, Ahlenius S: Further evidence for clozapine as a dopamine D1 receptor agonist. Eur J Pharmacol 307:27–31, 1996

Salmi P, Ahlenius S: Dihydrexidine produces hypothermia in rats via activation of dopamine D1 receptors. Neurosci Lett 236:57–59, 1997

Salmi P, Ahlenius S: Evidence for functional interactions between 5-HT 1A and 5-HT 2A receptors in rat thermoregulatory mechanisms. Pharmacol Toxicol 82:122–127, 1998

Salmi P, Jimenez S, Ahlenius S: Evidence for specific involvement of dopamine D-1 and D-2 receptors in regulation of body temperature in the rat. Eur J Pharmacol 236:395–400, 1993

Salmi P, Karlsson T, Ahlenius S: Antagonism by SCH 23390 of clozapine-induced hypothermia in the rat. Eur J Pharmacol 253:67–73, 1994

Samson-Fang I, Gooch J, Norlin C: Intrathecal baclofen withdrawal simulating neuroleptic malignant syndrome in a child with cerebral palsy. Dev Med Child Neurol 42:561–565, 2000

Sandyk R: L-dopa induced serotonin syndrome in a parkinsonian patient on bromocriptine (letter). J Clin Psychopharmacol 6:194–195, 1986

Sandyk R, Hurwitz MD: Toxic irreversible encephalopathy induced by lithium carbonate and haloperidol. S Afr Med J 64:875–876, 1983

Sangal R, Dimitrijevic R: Neuroleptic malignant syndrome: successful treatment with pancuronium. JAMA 254:2795–2796, 1985

Sansone MEG, Ziegler DK: Lithium neurotoxicity: a review of neuroleptic complications. Clin Neuropharmacol 8:242–248, 1985

Saran A, Addy O, Foliart RH, et al: Electroencephalographic changes and other indices of neurotoxicity with haloperidol-lithium therapy. Neuropsychobiology 20:152–157, 1989

Satinoff E: Neural organization and evolution of thermal regulation in mammals. Science 201:16–22, 1978

Sato T, Hara T, Takeichi M: A case of neuroleptic malignant syndrome with a history of general anesthesia. Human Psychopharmacology 7:351–353, 1992

Schafer JA: Body temperature regulation, in Essential Medical Physiology. Edited by Johnson LR. Philadelphia, PA, Lippincott-Raven, 1998, pp 815–824

Scheftner WA, Shulman RB: Treatment choice in neuroleptic malignant syndrome. Convulsive Therapy 8:267–279, 1992

Scheideggar W: Katatone Todesfalle in der Psychiatrischen Kinik von Zurich con 1900 bis 1928. Zeitschrift fur die Gesamte Neurol und Psychiatrie 120:587–649, 1929

Schibuk M, Schachter D: A role for catecholamines in the pathogenesis of neuroleptic malignant syndrome. Can J Psychiatry 31:66–69, 1986

Schneider C, Pedrosa-Gil F, Schneider M, et al: Intolerance to neuroleptics and susceptibility for malignant hyperthermia in a patient with proximal myotonic myopathy (PROMM) and schizophrenia. Neuromuscul Disord 12:31–35, 2002

Schou M: Long-lasting neurological sequelae after lithium intoxication. Acta Psychiatr Scand 70:594–602, 1984

Schrader GD: Neuroleptic malignant syndrome (letter). Med J Aust 69:367, 1982

Schuster CR, Lewis M, Seiden LS: Fenfluramine neurotoxicity. Psychopharmacol Bull 22:148–151, 1986

Schwartz JC, Diaz J, Pilon C, et al: Possible implications of dopamine D-3 receptor in schizophrenia and in antipsychotic drug actions. Brain Res Rev 31:277–287, 2000

Scott NR, Boulant JA: Dopamine effects on thermosensitive neurons in hypothalamic tissue slices. Brain Res 306:157–163, 1984

Screaton GR, Singer M, Cairns HS, et al: Hyperpyrexia and rhabdomyolysis after MDMA ("ecstasy") abuse (letter). Lancet 339:677–678, 1992

Sechi G, Agnetti V, Masuri R, et al: Risperidone, neuroleptic malignant syndrome and probable dementia with Lewy bodies. Prog Neuropsychopharmacol Biol Psychiatry 24:1043–1051, 2000

Sechi GP, Tanda F, Mutani R: Fatal hyperpyrexia after withdrawal of levodopa. Neurology 34:249–251, 1984

Sedivic V: [Psychoses endangering life]. Cesk Psychiatr 77:38–41, 1981

Seeman P: Antipsychotic drugs, dopamine receptors, and schizophrenia. Clin Neurosci Res 1:53–60, 2001

Seeman P, Tallerico T: Rapid release of antipsychotic drugs from dopamine D2 receptors: an explanation for low occupancy and early clinical relapse upon withdrawal of clozapine and quetiapine. Am J Psychiatry 156:876–884, 1999

Sellers EM, Roy ML, Martin PR, et al: Amphetamines, in Body Temperature: Regulation, Drug Effects and Therapeutic Implications. Edited by Lomax P, Schonbaum E. New York, Marcel Dekker, 1979, pp 461–498

Sellers J, Tyler P, Whitley A, et al: Neurotoxic effects of lithium with delayed rise in serum lithium levels. Br J Psychiatry 140:623–625, 1982

Semple DM, Ebmeier KP, Glabus MF, et al: Reduced *in vivo* binding to the seroto-nin transporter in the cerebral cortex of MDMA ('ecstasy') users. Psychol Med 175:63–69, 1999

Sewell DD, Jeste DU: Distinguishing neuroleptic malignant syndrome (NMS) from NMS-like acute medical illnesses: a study of 34 cases. J Neuropsychiatry Clin Neurosci 4:265–269, 1992

Shader RI, Greenblatt DJ: Uses and toxicity of belladonna alkaloids and synthetic anticholinergics. Seminars in Psychiatry 3:449–476, 1971

Shalev A, Munitz H: The neuroleptic malignant syndrome: agent and host interac-tion. Acta Psychiatr Scand 73:337–347, 1986

Shalev A, Aizenberg D, Hermesh H, et al: [Summer heat and the neuroleptic ma-lignant syndrome]. Harefuah 110:6–8, 1986

Shalev A, Hermesh H, Munitz H: The role of external heat load in triggering the neuroleptic malignant syndrome. Am J Psychiatry 145:110–111, 1988

Shalev A, Hermesh H, Munitz H: Mortality from neuroleptic malignant syndrome. J Clin Psychiatry 50:18–25, 1989

Sherman WR, Munsel LY, Gish BG, et al: Effects of systemically administered lith-ium on phosphoinositide metabolism in rat brain, kidney and testis. J Neuro-chem 44:798–807, 1985

Shibolet S, Lancaster MC, Danyon Y: Heat stroke: a review. Aviat Space Environ Med 47:280–301, 1976

Shields WD, Bray PF: A danger of haloperidol therapy in children. J Pediatr 88: 301–303, 1976

Shill HA, Stacey MA: Malignant catatonia secondary to sporadic encephalitis le-thargica (letter). J Neurol Neurosurg Psychiatry 69:402–403, 2000

Shimomura K, Hashimoto M, Mori J, et al: Role of brain amines in the fatal hyper-pyrexia caused by tranylcypromine in LiCl-pretreated rats. Jpn J Pharmacol 29:161–170, 1979

Shopsin B, Gershon S: Cogwheel rigidity related to lithium maintenance. Am J Psychiatry 132:536–538, 1975

Shopsin B, Small JG, Kellaus JJ, et al: Combining lithium and neuroleptics (letter). Am J Psychiatry 133:980–981, 1976

Shulack NR: Exhaustion syndrome in excited psychotic patients. Am J Psychiatry 102:466–475, 1946

Siegfried RN, Jacobsen L, Chabal C: Development of an acute withdrawal syn-drome following the cessation of intrathecal baclofen in a patient with spastic-ity. Anesthesiology 77:1048–1050, 1992

Silva RR, Munoz DM, Alpert M, et al: Neuroleptic malignant syndrome in children and adolescents. J Am Acad Child Adolesc Psychiatry 38:187–194, 1999

Simpson DM, Davis GC: Case report of neuroleptic malignant syndrome associ-ated with withdrawal from amantadine. Am J Psychiatry 141:796–797, 1984

Simpson GM, Branchey MH, Lee JH, et al: Lithium in tardive dyskinesia. Pharma-copsychiatry 9:76–80, 1976

Singarajah C, Lavies NG: An overdose of ecstasy: a role for dantrolene. Anaesthesia 47:686–687, 1992

Singerman B, Raheja R: Malignant catatonia—a continuing reality. Ann Clin Psychiatry 6:259–266, 1994

Singh TH: Neuroleptic malignant syndrome (letter). Br J Psychiatry 145:98, 1984

Skop BP, Finkelstein JF, Mareth TR, et al: The serotonin syndrome associated with paroxetine, an over-the-counter cold remedy and vascular disease. Am J Emerg Med 12:642–644, 1994

Small JG, Kellams JJ, Milstein V, et al: A placebo-controlled study of lithium combined with neuroleptics in chronic schizophrenic patients. Am J Psychiatry 132:1315–1317, 1975

Smilkstein MJ, Smolinske SC, Rumack BH: A case of MAO inhibitor/MDMA interaction: agony after ecstasy. J Toxicol Clin Toxicol 25:149–159, 1987

Smith B, Prockop DJ: Central nervous system effects of ingestion of L-tryptophan by normal subjects. N Engl J Med 267:1338–1341, 1962

Smith DF, Shimizu M, Schon M: Lithium absorption, distribution and clearance and body temperature in rats given lithium plus haloperidol. Pharmacology 15:337–340, 1977

Smith DL, Wenegrat BG: A case report of serotonin syndrome associated with combined nefazodone and fluoxetine (letter). J Clin Psychiatry 61:146, 2000

Smith LM, Peroutka SJ: Differential effects of 5-hydroxytryptamine$_{1A}$ selective drugs on the 5-HT behavioral syndrome. Pharmacol Biochem Behav 24:1513–1519, 1986

Snider RM, Fisher SK, Agranoff BW: Inositide-linked second messengers in the central nervous system, in Psychopharmacology: The Third Generation of Progress. Edited by Meltzer HY. New York, Raven, 1987, pp 317–324

Sobanski T, Bagli M, Laux G, et al: Serotonin syndrome after lithium add-on medication to paroxetine. Pharmacopsychiatry 30:106–107, 1997

Sokoloff P, Giros B, Martres MP, et al: Molecular cloning of and characterization of a novel dopamine receptor (D3) as a target for neuroleptics. Nature 347:146–151, 1990

Somers CJ, McLoughlin JV: Malignant hyperthermia in pigs: calcium ion uptake by mitochondria from skeletal muscle in susceptible animals given neuroleptic drugs and halothane. J Comp Pathol 92:191–195, 1982

Spigset O, Adielsson G: Combined serotonin syndrome and hyponatremia caused by a citalopram-buspirone interaction. Int Clin Psychopharmacol 12:61–63, 1997

Spigset O, Mjorndal T, Lovheim O: Serotonin syndrome caused by a moclobemide-clomipramine interaction (letter). BMJ 306:248, 1993

Spivak B, Maline DI, Vered Y, et al: Prospective evaluation of circulatory levels of catecholamines and serotonin in neuroleptic malignant syndrome. Acta Psychiatr Scand 102:226–230, 2000

Sporer KA: The serotonin syndrome: implicated drugs, pathophysiology and management. Drug Saf 13:94–104, 1995

Spring GK: EEG observations in confirming neurotoxicity (letter). Am J Psychiatry 136:1099–1100, 1979

Spring G, Frankel M: New data on lithium and haloperidol incompatibility. Am J Psychiatry 138:818–821, 1981

Stauder KH: Die todliche Katatonie. Archiv fur Psychiatrie und Nervenkrankheiten 102:614–634, 1934

Staunton DA, Magistretti PJ, Schoemaker WJ, et al: Effects of chronic lithium treatment on dopamine receptors in the rat corpus striatum, I: locomotor activity and behavioral supersensitivity. Brain Res 232:391–400, 1982a

Staunton DA, Magistretti PJ, Schoemaker WJ, et al: Effects of chronic lithium treatment on dopamine receptors in the rat corpus striatum, II: no effect on denervation or neuroleptic-induced supersensitivity. Brain Res 232:401–412, 1982b

Steele TE: Adverse reactions suggesting amoxapine-induced dopamine blockade. Am J Psychiatry 139:1500–1501, 1982

Sternbach H: The serotonin syndrome. Am J Psychiatry 148:705–713, 1991

Sternberg DE, Bowers MB Jr, Heninger GR, et al: Lithium prevents adaptation of brain dopamine systems to haloperidol in schizophrenic brains. Psychiatry Res 10:79–86, 1983

Stitt JT: Fever versus hyperthermia. Federation Proceedings 38:39–43, 1979

Stoudemire A, Luther JS: Neuroleptic malignant syndrome and neuroleptic-induced catatonia: differential diagnosis and treatment. Int J Psychiatry Med 14:57–63, 1984

Straker M: Neuroleptic malignant syndrome: fatalities associated with neuroleptic use and schizophrenia. Psychiatric Journal of the University of Ottawa 11:28–30, 1986

Strayhorn JM, Nash JL: Severe neurotoxicity despite "therapeutic" serum lithium levels. Diseases of the Nervous System 38:107–111, 1977

Sulpizio A, Fowler PJ, Macko E: Antagonism of fenfluramine-induced hyperthermia: a measure of central serotonin inhibition. Life Sci 22:1439–1446, 1978

Surmont DWA, Colardyn F, De Reuck J: Fatal complications of neuroleptic drugs: a clinico-pathological study of three cases. Acta Neurol Belg 84:75–83, 1984

Susman VL, Addonizio G: Reinduction of neuroleptic malignant syndrome by lithium. J Clin Psychopharmacol 7:339–341, 1987

Susman VL, Addonizio G: Recurrence of neuroleptic malignant syndrome: J Nerv Ment Dis 176:234–241, 1988

Suzuki A, Kondo T, Otani K, et al: Association of the TaqIA polymorphism of the dopamine D_2 receptor gene with predisposition to neuroleptic malignant syndrome. Am J Psychiatry 158:1714–1716, 2001

Swanson LW: An autoradiographic study of the efferent connections of the preoptic region of the rat. J Comp Neurol 167:227–256, 1976

Tang CP, Leung CM, Ungvari GS, et al: The syndrome of lethal catatonia. Singapore Med J 36:400–402, 1995

Tanii H, Taniguchi N, Niigawa H, et al: Development of an animal model for neuroleptic malignant syndrome: heat-exposed rabbits with haloperidol and atropine administration exhibit increased muscle activity, hyperthermia, and high serum creatine phosphokinase level. Brain Res 743:263–270, 1996

Tanvetyanon T, Dissin J, Selder UM: Hyperthermia and chronic pancerebellar syndrome after cocaine abuse. Arch Intern Med 161:608–610, 2001

Tarsy D: Neuroleptic-induced extrapyramidal reactions: classification, description, and diagnosis. Clin Neuropharmacol 6 (suppl 1):9–26, 1983

Taylor MA: Catatonia: a review of a behavioral neurologic syndrome. Neuropsychiatry Neuropsychol Behav Neurol 3:48–72, 1990

Taylor NE, Schwartz HI: Neuroleptic malignant syndrome following amoxapine overdose. J Nerv Ment Dis 176:249–251, 1988

Tenenbein M: The neuroleptic malignant syndrome: occurrence in a 15-year-old boy and recovery with bromocriptine therapy. Pediatric Neuroscience 12:161–164, 1986

Tesio I, Porta GL, Messa E: Cerebellar syndrome in lithium poisoning: a case of partial recovery (letter). J Neurol Neurosurg Psychiatry 50:235, 1987

Thase ME, Shostak M: Rhabdomyolysis complicating rapid intramuscular neuroleptization. J Clin Psychopharmacol 4:46–48, 1984

Theoharides TC, Harris RS, Weckstein D: Neuroleptic malignant-like syndrome due to cyclobenzaprine (letter)? J Clin Psychopharmacol 15:79–81, 1995

Thierry AM, Tassin JP, Blanc G, et al: Selective activation of the mesocortical dopamine system by stress. Nature 263:242–244, 1976

Thomas CJ: Brain damage with lithium/haloperidol (letter). Br J Psychiatry 134:552, 1979

Thomas K, Rajeev KK, Abraham CC, et al: Management of neuroleptic malignant syndrome. Journal of Association of Physicians of India 41:91–93, 1993

Tignol J, Meggle D: Syndrome malin, in Dictionnaire des Neuroleptiques. Edited by Colonna L, Petit M, Lepine J-P. Paris, France, JB Baillere, 1989, pp 366–371

Torline RL: Extreme hyperpyrexia associated with central anticholinergic syndrome. Anesthesiology 76:470–471, 1992

Trivedi S: Psychiatric symptoms in carcinoid syndrome. J Indian Med Assoc 82:292–294, 1984

Troller JN, Sachdev PS: Electroconvulsive treatment of neuroleptic malignant syndrome: a review and report of cases. Aust N Z J Psychiatry 33:650–659, 1999

Tsutsumi Y, Yamamoto K, Hata S, et al: Incidence of "typical cases" and "incomplete cases" of neuroleptic malignant syndrome and their epidemiological study. Japanese Journal of Psychiatry 48:789–799, 1994

Tsutsumi Y, Yamamoto K, Matsunra S, et al: The treatment of neuroleptic malignant syndrome using dantrolene sodium. Psychiatry Clin Neurosci 52:433–438, 1998

Tupin JP, Schuller AB: Lithium and haloperidol incompatibility reviewed. Psychiatric Journal of the University of Ottawa 3:245–251, 1978

Turner E, Reddy H: Iron in neuroleptic malignant syndrome (letter). Lancet 338:820, 1991

Turner MR, Gainsborough N: Neuroleptic malignant-like syndrome after abrupt withdrawal of baclofen. J Psychopharmacol 15:61–63, 2001

Tyrer P, Alexander MS, Regan A: An extrapyramidal syndrome after lithium therapy. Br J Psychiatry 136:191–194, 1980

Ueda M, Hamamoto M, Nagayama H, et al: Susceptibility to neuroleptic malignant syndrome in Parkinson's disease. Neurology 52:777–781, 1999

Ueda M, Hamamoto M, Nagayama H, et al: Biochemical alterations during medication withdrawal in Parkinson's disease with and without neuroleptic malignant-like syndrome. J Neurol Neurosurg Psychiatry 71:111–113, 2001

Ueno S, Otani K, Kaneko S, et al: Cytochrome P-450 2D6 gene polymorphism is not associated with neuroleptic malignant syndrome. Biol Psychiatry 40:72–74, 1996

Ulus IH, Kiran BK, Ozkurt S: Involvement of central dopamine in the hyperthermia in rats produced by d-amphetamine. Pharmacology 13:309–316, 1975

Unger J, Decaux G, L'Hermite M: Rhabdomyolysis, acute renal failure, endocrine alterations and neurological sequelae in a case of lithium self poisoning. Acta Clin Belg 37:216–223, 1982

Van de Kelft E, De Hert M, Heytens L, et al: Management of lethal catatonia with dantrolene sodium. Crit Care Med 19:1449–1451, 1991

van Harten PN, Kemperman CJF: Organic amnestic disorder: a long-term sequel after neuroleptic malignant syndrome. Biol Psychiatry 29:407–410, 1991

van Kammen DP, Marder SR: Clozapine, in Comprehensive Textbook of Psychiatry, 6th Edition. Edited by Kaplan HI, Sadock BJ. Baltimore, MD, Williams & Wilkins, 1995, pp 1979–1987

Velamoor VR, Fernando MLD, Williamson P: Incipient neuroleptic malignant syndrome. Br J Psychiatry 156:581–584, 1990

Velamoor VR, Norman RMG, Caroff SN, et al: Progression of symptoms in neuroleptic malignant syndrome. J Nerv Ment Dis 182:168–173, 1994

Velamoor VR, Swamy GN, Parmar RS, et al: Management of suspected neuroleptic malignant syndrome. Can J Psychiatry 40:545–550, 1995

Venkatachari SAT, Pagala M, Herzlich B, et al: Effect of cocaine on neuromusclar function in isolated phrenic nerve diaphragm of mouse. FASEB J 2:A1138, 1988

Verma A, Kulkarni SK: Differential role of dopamine receptor subtypes in thermoregulation and stereotypic behavior in naïve and reserpinized rats. Archives Internationales de Pharmacodynamie et de Therapie 324:17–32, 1993

Vigran IM: Dangerous potentiation of meperidine hydrochloride by pargyline hydrochloride. JAMA 187:953–954, 1964

Vincent FM, Zimmerman JE, Van Haren J: Neuroleptic malignant syndrome complicating closed head injury. Neurosurgery 18:190–193, 1986

Vizi ES, Illes P, Ronai A, et al: The effect of lithium on acetylcholine release and synthesis. Neuropharmacology 11:521–530, 1972

Voigt MM, Uhl GR: Neurotransmitter receptor alterations, in Handbook of Parkinson's Disease. Edited by Koller WC. New York, Marcel Dekker, 1987, pp 253–266

Volkow ND, Harper A, Munnisteri D, et al: AIDS and catatonia (letter). J Neurol Neurosurg Psychiatry 50:104, 1987 von Knorring L, Smigan L, Perris C, et al: Lithium and neuroleptic drugs in combination—effect on lithium RBC/plasma ratio. International Pharmacopsychiatry 17:287–292, 1982

von Muhlendahl KE, Krienke EG: Fenfluramine poisoning. Clin Toxicol 14:97–106, 1979

Wachtel TJ, Steele GH, Day JA: Natural history of fever following seizure. Arch Intern Med 147:1153–1155, 1987

Walenga RW, Opas EE, Feinstein MB: Differential effects of calmodulin antagonists on phospholipase A2 and C in thrombin-stimulated platelets. J Biol Chem 256:12523–12528, 1981

Wappler F, Fiege M, Schulte am Esch J: Pathophysiological role of the serotonin system in malignant hyperthermia. Br J Anaesth 87:793–797, 2001

Watson JD, Ferguson C, Hinds CJ, et al: Exertional heat stroke induced by amphetamine analogues: does dantrolene have a place? Anaesthesia 48:1057–1060, 1993

Weiden PJ: Ziprasidone: a new atypical antipsychotic. Journal of Psychiatric Practice 7:145–153, 2001

Weinberger DR, Kelly MJ: Catatonia and malignant syndrome: a possible complication of neuroleptic administration. J Nerv Ment Dis 165:263–268, 1977

Weiner AL: Meperidine as a potential cause of serotonin syndrome in the emergency department. Acad Emerg Med 6:156–158, 1999

Weiner AL, Tilden FF Jr, McKay CA Jr: Serotonin syndrome: case report and review of the literature. Conn Med 61:717–721, 1997

Weiner LA, Smythe M, Cisek J: Serotonin syndrome secondary to phenelzine-venlafaxine interaction. Pharmacotherapy 18:399–403, 1998

Weis J: On the hyperthermic response to d-amphetamine in the decapitated rat. Life Sci 13:475–484, 1973

Weiss DM: Serotonin syndrome in Parkinson's disease. J Am Board Fam Pract 8:400–402, 1995

Weller M, Kornhuber J: A rationale for NMDA receptor antagonist therapy of the neuroleptic malignant syndrome. Med Hypotheses 38:329–333, 1992a

Weller M, Kornhuber J: Lyell syndrome and lethal catatonia: a case for ECT (letter). Am J Psychiatry 149:1114, 1992b

Weller M, Kornhuber J: Serum iron levels in neuroleptic malignant syndrome (letter). Biol Psychiatry 34:123, 1993

Wells AJ, Sommi RW, Crismon ML: Neuroleptic rechallenge after neuroleptic malignant syndrome: case report and literature review. Drug Intelligence and Clinical Pharmacy 22:475–480, 1988

White DAC: Catatonia and the neuroleptic malignant syndrome: a single entity? Br J Psychiatry 161:558–560, 1992

White DAC, Robins AH: Catatonia: harbinger of the neuroleptic malignant syndrome. Br J Psychiatry 158:419–421, 1991

White DAC, Robins AH: An analysis of 17 catatonic patients diagnosed with neuroleptic malignant syndrome. CNS Spectrums 5:58–65, 2000

White SR, Obradovic T, Imiel KM, et al: The effects of methylene dioxymetham-phetamine (MDMA, "ecstasy") on monoaminergic neurotransmission in the central nervous system. Prog Neurobiol 49:455–479, 1996

Williams K, MacPherson R: Reintroduction of antipsychotics in a patient with clo-zapine-induced neuroleptic malignant syndrome. Irish Journal of Psychologi-cal Medicine 14:147–148, 1997

Wirtshafter D, Asin KE, Kent EW: Nucleus accumbens lesions reduce amphet-amine hyperthermia but not hyperactivity. Eur J Pharmacol 51:449–452, 1978

Wise TN: Heatstroke in three chronic schizophrenics: case reports and clinical considerations. Compr Psychiatry 14:263–267, 1973

Woodbury MM, Woodbury MA: Neuroleptic-induced catatonia as a stage in the progression toward neuroleptic malignant syndrome. J Am Acad Child Ado-lesc Psychiatry 31:1161–1164, 1992

Wooten GF: Neurochemistry, in Handbook of Parkinson's Disease. Edited by Kol-ler WC. New York, Marcel Dekker, 1987, pp 237–253

Yamawaki S, Lai H, Horita A: Dopaminergic and serotonergic mechanisms of ther-moregulation: mediation of thermal effects of apomorphine and dopamine. J Pharmacol Exp Ther 227:383–388, 1983

Yamawaki S, Yano E, Terakawa N, et al: On the results of a nationwide survey on neuroleptic malignant syndrome. Hiroshima Journal of Anesthesia 24 (suppl 19):52–67, 1988

Yamawaki S, Kato T, Yano E: Studies on pathogenesis of neuroleptic malignant syn-drome: effect of dantrolene on serotonin release in rat hypothalamus. Hi-roshima Journal of Anesthesia 26:45–52, 1990a

Yamawaki S, Yano E, Uchitomi Y: Analysis of 497 cases of neuroleptic malignant syndrome in Japan. Hiroshima Journal of Anesthesia 26:35–44, 1990b

Yamawaki S, Morio M, Kazamutsuri G, et al: Clinical evaluation and effective usage of dantrolene sodium in neuroleptic malignant syndrome. Kiso to Rinsyou (Clinical Reports) 27:1045–1066, 1993

Yamawaki Y, Ogawa N: Successful treatment of levodopa-induced neuroleptic ma-lignant syndrome (NMS) and disseminated intravascular coagulation (DIC) in a patient with Parkinson's disease. Intern Med 31:1298–1302, 1992

Yassa R, Archer J, Cordozo S: The long-term effect of lithium carbonate on tardive dyskinesia. Can J Psychiatry 29:36–37, 1984

Yehuda S, Wurtman RJ: Dopaminergic neurons in the nigro-striatal and mesolim-bic pathways: mediation of specific effects of d-amphetamine. Eur J Pharmacol 30:154–158, 1975

Yoshikawa H, Oda Y, Sakajiri K, et al: Pure akinesia manifested neuroleptic malig-nant syndrome: a clinical variant of progressive supranuclear palsy. Acta Neu-ropathol (Berl) 93:306–309, 1997

Zalis EG, Kaplan G, Lundberg GD, et al: Acute lethality of the amphetamines in dogs and its antagonism by curare. Proc Soc Exp Biol Med 118:577–561, 1965

Zalis EG, Lundberg GD, Knutson RA: The pathophysiology of acute amphet-amine poisoning with pathologic considerations. J Pharmacol Exp Ther 158: 115–127, 1967

Zelman S, Guillan R: Heatstroke in phenothiazine-treated patients: a report of three fatalities. Am J Psychiatry 126:1787–1790, 1970

Zimmerschied JA, Harry B: Serotonin syndrome in a prisoner. J Forensic Sci 43: 208–209, 1998

Index

*Page numbers printed in **boldface type** refer to tables or figures.*